Therapeutic Hypothermia After Cardiac Arrest

Justin B. Lundbye
Editor

Therapeutic Hypothermia After Cardiac Arrest

Clinical Application and Management

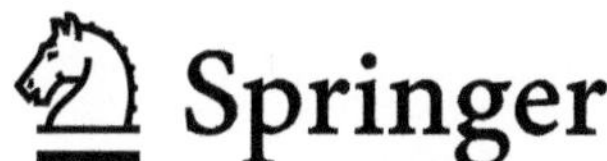

Editor
Justin B. Lundbye, M.D. FACC
Division of Cardiology
Hospital of Central Connecticut
New Britain, CT
USA

University of Connecticut
School of Medicine
Farmington, CT,
USA

ISBN 978-1-4471-2950-9 ISBN 978-1-4471-2951-6 (eBook)
DOI 10.1007/978-1-4471-2951-6
Springer Dordrecht Heidelberg New York London

Library of Congress Control Number: 2012942605

Printed on acid-free paper

Springer is part of Springer Science+Business Media (www.springer.com)

This book is dedicated to my wife, Kristen, my children, Elana and Jude, and my mother, Anne

Foreword

Therapeutic hypothermia is the major breakthrough for post-resuscitation care in our generation. Currently, it is the only treatment available to provide neuropreservation when applied after a critical event, i.e., cardiac arrest. Nonetheless, surveys reveal that less than 50 % of all medical centers in the United States provide this life-sparing therapy.

This book is a well-done summary of the major issues that surround therapeutic hypothermia provided to post-resuscitated patients. In a field clearly in flux, the book's up-to-date chapters provide useful information on how to start a therapeutic hypothermia program, who should be considered for such a treatment, what cooling methods are currently available, and the potential cautions particularly concerning therapeutic hypothermia and pharmacologic interactions, as well as other potential adverse effects.

This volume is well written with specific details that can be extremely helpful in beginning a therapeutic hypothermia program. It is truly a welcomed edition for all those who recognize the need to begin providing this life-saving and central nervous system–sparing therapy for post-cardiac arrest patients.

Tucson, Arizona

Karl B. Kern, M.D., FACC, FAHA, FSCAI, FACP

Preface

When I began my role as CICU director at Hartford Hospital in 2006, the hospital had yet to institute a TH protocol, though there had been much discussion and, under the direction of Dr. Jeff Kluger, the framework had been laid. Using the program established at the Hospital of the University of Pennsylvania as a guide, HH treated its first patient in early 2007. As our experience grew, not only did the benefits of TH present themselves to me, but I also became acutely aware of the lack of information on the topic and the necessity of furthering research to make others aware of it as well.

For out of hospital cardiac arrests, the AHA currently recommends TH at Level I for shockable rhythms and Level IIb for nonshockable rhythms. Despite these recommendations, TH is still underutilized in these patient populations, perhaps because of an unfamiliarity and insufficient information on how to initiate it.

The purpose of this book is to provide an evidence based approach to identifying and managing cardiac arrest patients who are appropriate for TH. Aimed at ER physicians and staff, intensivists, mid-level practitioners, nursing staff, and EMS, this comprehensive manual answers the how, why, and when to initiate therapy. It should provide the reader with the necessary tools to design, apply, and successfully manage a TH program at their institution.

Acknowledgments

This book would not have been possible without the involvement of many people.

I would first like to thank each of the contributors who gave their expertise to ensure that this guide is as comprehensive as possible. I would especially like to thank those who worked within very short time lines despite their own very busy schedules. I also want to recognize that many of the contributors took time away from their families and loved ones to participate in this work. I am grateful for and appreciate your willingness to do so.

I would also like to thank Dr. Gary Heller, whose accomplishments are too many to list. He has been a consummate leader, mentor, and friend for many years in matters both professional and personal. His is a path I am honored to follow.

Special thanks go to Kathryn Kircher, who has worked tirelessly by my side since 2007. Her efforts steer me in the right direction and smooth the bumps in the road along the way. Thank you!

Finally, I would like to thank my children, Elana and Jude, for their support and understanding while I conquer my goals. I also want to thank my wife and friend Kristen for her support in making this book a possibility. Her skills, patience, and attention to detail have been invaluable.

Contents

Contributors

Benjamin S. Abella, M.D. Department of Emergency Medicine, Center for Resuscitation Science, University of Pennsylvania, Philadelphia, PA, USA

Edgar Argulian, M.D. Division of Cardiology, Department of Medicine, New York, NY, USA

Renata Barbosa, RN Division of Cardiology, Department of Medicine, New York, NY, USA

William L. Baker, Pharm.D., BCPS Department of Pharmacy and Medicine, University of Connecticut, Schools of Pharmacy and Medicine, Storrs, Farmington, CT, USA

M. Ross Bullock, M.D. Ph.D. Department of Neurosurgery, Miami Project to Cure Paralysis, University of Miami Miller School of Medicine, Miami, FL, USA

W. Dalton Dietrich, Ph.D. Department of Neurosurgery, Miami Project to Cure Paralysis, University of Miami Miller School of Medicine, Miami, FL, USA

David Erlinge, M.D., Ph.D. Department of Cardiology, Lund University, Skane University Hospital, Lund, Sweden

Lisa Hawksworth, MSN, RN, NE-BC Cardiovascular Services, Mary Washington Healthcare, Fredericksburg, VA, USA

Eyal Herzog, M.D. Division of Cardiology, Department of Medicine, New York, NY, USA

Cara Klajbor, M.D. Department of Neurology, Hartford Hospital, Hartford, CT, USA

Justin B. Lundbye, M.D. FACC Division of Cardiology, Department of Medicine, Hartford, CT, USA

University of Connecticut School of Medicine, Farmington, CT, USA

Xia Luo, M.D. Clinical Education, ZOLL, Sunnyvale, CA, USA

Sanjeev U. Nair, MBBS, M.D., FACP Division of Cardiology, Department of Medicine, Hartford, CT, USA

University of Connecticut School of Medicine, Farmington, CT, USA

Matthew W. Parker, M.D. Division of Cardiology, Department of Medicine, Hartford, CT, USA

University of Connecticut School of Medicine, Farmington, CT, USA

Kelly Sawyer, M.D., M.S. Department of Emergency Medicine, Oakland University William Beaumont School of Medicine, Royal Oak, MI, USA

Erica Schuyler, M.D. Department of Neurology, Hartford Hospital, Hartford, CT, USA

Department of Medicine, University of Connecticut School of Medicine, Farmington, CT, USA

Janet Shapiro, M.D. Division of Pulmonary and Critical care, Department of Medicine, New York, NY, USA

Sarah K. Wallace Department of Emergency Medicine, Center for Resuscitation Science, Hospital of the University of Pennsylvania, Philadelphia, PA, USA

Johns Hopkins University School of Medicine, Baltimore, MD, USA

Shoji Yokobori, M.D., Ph.D. Department of Neurosurgery, Nippon Medical School, Tokyo, Japan

Department of Neurosurgery, Miami Project to Cure Paralysis, University of Miami Miller School of Medicine, Miami, FL, USA

1 Introduction

Kelly Sawyer

We are here to add what we can to, not to get what we can from, life.
– Sir William Osler

Reflections

In 2010 I attended my first Resuscitation Science Symposium (ReSS) in Chicago, Illinois. As an Emergency Cardiac Care Fellow at Virginia Commonwealth University Medical Center (VCUMC), I had begun to ask questions about cardiac arrest and the use of therapeutic hypothermia. At VCUMC, the Advanced Resuscitation Cooling Therapeutic Intensive Care (ARCTIC) team provided a multidisciplinary approach to patients admitted after cardiac arrest. They had improved survival and neurological outcomes with comprehensive post-resuscitation care but many questions remained.

ReSS, which accompanies and precedes the annual American Heart Association (AHA) meeting, brought both cardiac and trauma resuscitation specialists together to share ideas. I was fortunate to attend the Young Investigator dinner, at which many successful investigators were willing to share experience and give advice to those of us aspiring to also pursue careers in resuscitation research. I found myself sitting next to Dr. James Jude, who was in attendance with Dr. Guy Knickerbocker to be honored with the Lifetime Achievement Award in Cardiac Resuscitation Science.

This year was the 50th Anniversary of the discovery and description by James Jude, Guy Knickerbocker, and William Kouwenhoven of closed chest cardiac massage [1]. They had worked together many years earlier at Johns Hopkins University and one day made, according to Dr. Jude, "a chance observation." Known most commonly as cardiopulmonary resuscitation, or CPR, it is an intervention that has since saved thousands of people. It changed the way the world approached sudden cardiac arrest, since "anyone, anywhere" [1] could initiate resuscitation for those "hearts (and brains) too good to die" [2, 3].

Several young investigators were interested in measuring the quality of CPR, establishing systems of care for cardiac arrest, improving outcomes with therapeutic hypothermia, and translating research from the laboratory to the bedside. The science we discussed and celebrated that weekend was cutting edge, bringing international researchers together for a common goal: to impact quality of life for those faced with otherwise imminent death from traumatic injury or cardiopulmonary arrest. And ironically, that science would also restore my life in the following year.

I have a unique perspective as both researcher and patient. Just before my fellowship ended, I collapsed from a massive pulmonary embolism. I was walking from the parking garage and suddenly became incredibly short of breath. Though I was a relatively active person and healthy, the chest pressure left me breathless.

K. Sawyer, M.D., MS
Department of Emergency Medicine, Oakland University William Beaumont School of Medicine, Royal Oak, MI, USA
e-mail: ksawyer6@yahoo.com

J.B. Lundbye (ed.), *Therapeutic Hypothermia After Cardiac Arrest*,
DOI 10.1007/978-1-4471-2951-6_1, © Springer-Verlag London 2012

I tried to just sit down, because my head was fuzzy. I knew I was about to pass out, but gravity took over. Fortunately bystanders were not afraid to come to my side, and I received quick assistance. The two nurses identified me from my pager, as I was only answering intermittent questions. Given the location in the hospital, EMS providers were called. At the same time, the Emergency Department (ED) was notified and my colleague rushed to help, gleaning only limited information from what I was able to communicate to him.

Approximately 3 weeks earlier, I had undergone arthroscopy for a torn meniscus. I had had some calf pain about 1 week post-operatively, and while I was also taking oral contraceptive pills (OCPs), the pain eventually resolved. I attributed it to a muscle strain related to limited range of motion and my need for physical therapy. I had even been working my shifts in the Emergency Department and completed my Master's Degree requirements. I do not recall any other obvious sign to portend the events that followed.

I was emergently transferred to the ED, where my own colleagues stepped up to care for one of their own. I was hypoxic and clinically too unstable for CT scanning. However, prompt Cardiology consultation and limited bedside echocardiography showed severe right heart strain and intr-atrial clot. Though full dose heparin and thrombolytics were given without hesitation, I continued to deteriorate. Cardiothoracic Surgery was present and ready to initiate ECMO but instead went straight to the operating room (OR) for cardiopulmonary bypass. Total time from collapse to the OR was about 45 min.

After emergent embolectomy, I was maintained under therapeutic hypothermia, just as I had provided to other patients – for all the same benefits this book will discuss. I awoke in the Cardiac Surgery ICU with lines and tubes I had no memory of being placed. My colleagues gave me the best chance for full recovery, and I surprised many, being discharged home just 2 weeks later. The comprehensive care by specialists in Emergency/Resuscitation Medicine, Cardiology, Cardiothoracic Surgery, and Critical Care was a successful effort that revealed the full potential for multidisciplinary collaboration among experts.

The guidelines for post-resuscitation care are now at the forefront of research efforts, and my story not only supports the expanding scope for therapeutic hypothermia but also highlights the hopeful possibility for Science in the future. It is with great pleasure resuscitation that I introduce you to the modern history of therapeutic hypothermia and how it has come to be used for improving cardiopulmonary-cerebral survival after cardiac arrest.

By medicine life may be prolong'd, yet death / Will seize the Doctor too.

– William Shakespeare

The Problem

Medicine and Science have actually seen many successes in the last century or two [4]. From pasteurization, sterilization, and vaccination to seat belts, helmets, and condoms, public health has had a major influence on morbidity and mortality around the world. Furthermore, with the discovery of antibiotics in the early twentieth century and efforts to provide safe water, food, and workplaces, the overall life expectancy in the United States has increased dramatically (Fig. 1.1) [5], while the death rate continues to fall (Fig. 1.2) [6]. Infant mortality has also decreased, a result attributable to initiatives encouraging immunization, good hand-washing, and oral rehydration.

Recent 2012 AHA statistics support a 30.6% [7] decline in the death rate related to cardiovascular disease and stroke in the US, though the prevalence of diabetes and obesity are worsening in all age groups. Yet, not since the discovery of CPR and external defibrillation in 1960 [1] has an intervention had a major impact on the natural history of sudden cardiac arrest [8]; that is until the recent emphasis on post-resuscitation care, including the use of therapeutic hypothermia.

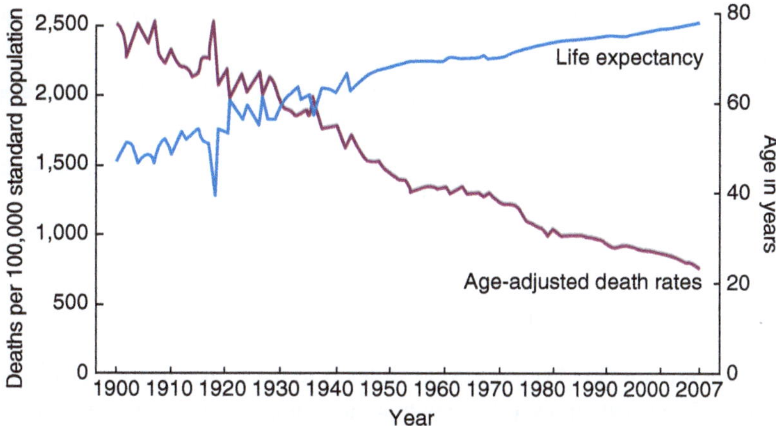

Fig. 1.1 Life expectancy & age-adjusted death rates: US, 1900–2007 [5]

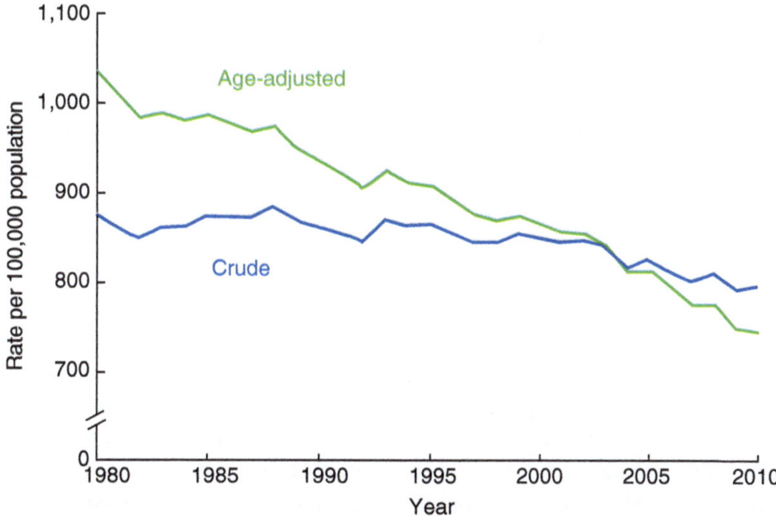

Fig. 1.2 Crude & age-adjusted death rates: US, 1980–2009 [6]

Sudden Death World Wide

Worldwide, causes of sudden death vary [9]. In Europe and the United States, ischemic heart disease is the most common cause of adult cardiac arrest. But outside of these areas, trauma, drowning, and infectious etiologies are very important causes of death. For children, diarrhea, pneumonia, malnutrition, trauma, drowning, and asphyxia are more common than cardiac etiologies of sudden death. Numerous non-profit organizations work to build infrastructure, teach principles of "germ theory", and institute local public health programs in areas where simple education can make a tremendous impact on morbidity and mortality. As urbanization increases, however, cardiovascular disease will likely become a more important factor on the list of causes of sudden death around the world.

Cardiac Arrest: United States

Despite efforts to raise awareness and affect change in modifiable risk factors, cardiovascular

Fig. 1.3 American Heart Association, chain of survival [14]

- Immediate recognition and activation of the emergency response system by calling 911
- Early cardiopulmonary resuscitation (CPR), emphasizing chest compressions only for bystanders
- Rapid defibrillation, using an automated external defibrillator (AED) if available or manual device by professionals
- Effective advanced life support by emergency care providers
- Integrated post-cardiac arrest care

disease remains the leading cause of death in the United States [9], and sudden death is most often related to ischemic heart disease. Each year, approximately 380,000 people in the United States suffer from non-traumatic out-of-hospital cardiac arrest (OOH-CA) [7]. Of those, about 60% are treated by EMS personnel and 23% have an initial shockable rhythm. An average of 11.4% of OOH-CA patients, treated by EMS, survives to hospital discharge [7].

In children under the age of 18, an estimated 8.6% of OOH-CA patients survive to discharge [7]. In athletes, about half (56%) were attributed to cardiovascular disease, including 11% in females and 82% during physical competition or training. Etiologies include long QT, short QT, and Brugada syndromes and structural anomalies, most commonly hypertrophic cardiomyopathy or aberrant coronary arteries. Approximately 1 in 500 individuals have hypertrophic cardiomyopathy, and the risk of sudden death increases with increasing left ventricular wall thickness [7].

According to Get With the Guidelines – Resuscitation (GWTG-R), approximately 200,000 patients a year suffer an in-hospital cardiac arrest (IHCA) [10]. For adults and children, roughly 23.1% and 35.0%, respectively, survive to discharge [7]. As in children, the focus for improving outcomes for patients with IHCA has been on the "chain of prevention" [11]. Methods to this end in children include prevention of injury by wearing seatbelts and bike helmets, supervising swimming pools and kitchen stoves, and securing firearms and small objects that are prone to cause choking. In-hospital, efforts have been focused on the effectiveness of rapid response teams (RRTs) and increased monitoring of patients [12]. Much like in the out-of-hospital setting, early recognition and defibrillation, as well as comprehensive post-resuscitation care, are recommended to maximize survival [11].

A small study of adults revealed that the majority of them were familiar with what actions to take in the event of a medical emergency, and about 98% recognized the purpose of an automated external defibrillator (AED) [7]. However, other studies have been discouraging, suggesting that even with knowledge, lay persons are often reluctant to intervene in the acute setting. Mass outreach aims to educate the public regarding the signs and symptoms of sudden cardiac arrest and to dissolve barriers to bystander CPR, and as of 2008, the AHA recommended hands-only CPR for lay bystanders of witnessed cardiac arrest [13]. Since more than half of OOH-CA's are witnessed, bystanders are crucial players in the "chain of survival" (Fig. 1.3) [14]. Groups such as the AHA, Sudden Cardiac Arrest Foundation, and Sudden Cardiac Arrest Association, as well as more local, grass-roots efforts, are committed to community outreach and education.

All progress is experimental.

– John Jay Chapman

Early Experimentation: 1940s–1950s

Early modern investigation into hypothermia as a tool and medical therapy stemmed from neurosurgeon, Dr. Temple Fay, who induced hypothermia to alleviate pain in a cancer patient [15, 16]. In the 1940s, he and colleagues employed hypothermia for approximately 24 h in patients as a possible means to decrease cancer progression [15, 17]. While there was no observed effect on cancer cell division as a result of induced hypothermia, the patients seemed to tolerate it well. Later, they reported on observations of improved outcomes in severe head injury patients treated with hypothermia [15, 17].

Fay is credited with the first clinical use of hypothermia, including the development of the first cooling blanket [17]. His work inspired researchers to further experiment with the use of hypothermia in other settings, such as cardiac and neurosurgery [18], traumatic brain injury, stroke, acute myocardial infarction, and spinal cord injury. For discussion purposes, protective hypothermia is initiated prior to injury or ischemia; preservative hypothermia is initiated during injury; and resuscitative hypothermia, also known today as therapeutic hypothermia, is induced post-insult or injury.

The Cardiac Surgery Experience: Protective-Preservative Hypothermia

In 1950, Bigelow et al. [19] explored the use of hypothermia as a cerebral protectant during cardiac surgery in dogs. They used a target temperature of 20°C and had modest favorable outcomes upon rewarming. They further extended their research to monkeys and groundhogs [20] in order to observe the effects of an even lower goal temperature on other mammals, including one capable of hibernation. The target temperature for the monkeys was 16–19°C and the goal for the groundhogs was 2.5–5°C. In 1953, Bigelow and McBirnie [20] reported their results, including the successful revival of 12/13 monkeys and 5/6 groundhogs. Interestingly their other observations included the incidence of infection in these animals, possibly related to imperfect asepsis technique; the improved cold tolerance in younger animals; and the applicability of continuous EEG monitoring during induction and rewarming to monitor the effects of brain activity. This early work on animals led to advanced application of induced hypothermia for human cardiovascular surgery.

In humans, moderate hypothermia (28–32°C) began as an adjunct to closed cardiac surgery in the correction of cyanotic congenital heart disease in the 1940s. Surface methods were used to provide the therapy, aiming to decrease metabolic demand and oxygen requirements, in patients already experiencing oxygen debt, and decrease complications related to anesthesia. Still, closed techniques for cardiac surgery were not ideal, and in the early 1950s, surgeons investigated deep hypothermia (20–28°C) as a means to perform open heart procedures. Hypothermia was not just an aid at this stage but a reversible method to allow in-flow stasis and create a temporary bloodless field. The colder temperatures allowed a longer duration for operation under deprivation conditions (i.e. minutes of in-flow stasis), but as the depth of hypothermia increased, so did the risk for terminal fibrillation and coagulopathy.

As a consequence, in the late 1950s the limitations of time restriction and complication led to the development of extra-corporeal circulation machines. Known as the "heart-lung machine" or more recently cardiopulmonary bypass, a.k.a. "the pump", the possibility for extra-corporeal support alleviated the restriction on in-flow stasis time and opened the door for increasingly complex procedures. Once again hypothermia was an adjunct to cardiac surgery, and some speculated that with time and increasingly efficient machines, hypothermic therapy in cardiovascular surgery would become obsolete [21]. Others, especially when operating on adult patients, continued to use hypothermia for its protective-preservative value, believing that moderate hypothermia was needed for benefit.

Translational Research: Resuscitative Hypothermia After Cardiac Arrest

Early investigation into the use of resuscitative hypothermia, after sudden cardiac arrest or global ischemia, was first reported in the 1950s, though reliable animal models for cardiac arrest were lacking. In 1954, Rosomoff and Holaday [22] reported the proportional decrease in both cerebral oxygen consumption and cerebral blood flow with decreasing body temperature in dogs. Rosomoff and

Gilbert [23] later published results regarding the reduction in normal brain volume (by about 4%) under hypothermic conditions. Importantly, they further confirmed findings by Bigelow [19] that shivering increased both venous and cerebrospinal fluid pressures, necessitating adequate anesthesia during induction, even though global neurological dysfunction may be evident. These observations into the effects of hypothermia on the normal central nervous system, along with case reports on the benefits of hypothermia in patients with head injury [17], helped propose the leap to the use of induced hypothermia after injury and ischemia.

An important animal study in 1958, Zimmerman and Spencer [24] presented their results on the improved survival with resuscitative hypothermia after 10 min of cardiac arrest in dogs. A total of 14 were cooled with hypothermia (31–33°C) for 24–48 h and 57% survived. In contrast, only 25% of the normothermic dogs survived. Two pioneering papers were published on the clinical use of hypothermia after cardiac arrest about the same time.

Williams and Spencer [25] reported on four patients, each who suffered cardiac arrest outside of the operating room for approximately 5 min and were cooled for between 24 and 72 h at 30–34°C. All of them survived, three with no residual neurological deficit. Benson et al. [26] published the results of a small controlled study in 1959, wherein they successfully resuscitated 19 patients from cardiac arrest, 12 who were cooled and 7 who were not. Therapy was implemented to a temperature of 30–32°C, for a duration based on clinical judgment and signs of improvement. The survival rate in the hypothermia group was 50% versus 14% in the control group. While certainly a small sample with variable baseline characteristics, these results are reminiscent of recent investigations that have more firmly changed the practice of resuscitative hypothermia, some 40 years later.

Clinical Dormancy: 1960s–1970s

Clinical application was essentially abandoned for the observation of cardiac irritability and ventricular fibrillation with the use of hypothermia at temperatures below 30°C, at temperature thought to be necessary for optimal protection. Concerns for increased infection rates with pneumonia and bacteremia, as well as potential for bleeding, were risky enough to halt all but some animal model research during this time [16, 27].

Nevertheless, Dr. Peter Safar, who became the Chair of the Department of Anesthesia at the University of Pittsburgh in 1961, was a proponent of using hypothermia and included it in his cardiopulmonary-cerebral resuscitation sequence at that time. In many circles, he is renowned as the "Father of Modern Resuscitation" and credited as the developer of the "ABC's of Cardiopulmonary Resuscitation" [28]. He spent approximately 20 years in Pittsburgh before establishing the International Resuscitation Research Center, where he and colleagues would investigate the benefit of mild hypothermia (32–34°C) and revive the clinical use of resuscitative hypothermia in the lab.

> *Every great advance in science has issued from a new audacity of imagination.*
>
> *– John Dewey*

Research Resurgence: 1980s–1990s

Important Animal Studies

Resuscitation research resurfaced in the 1980s and 1990s (Fig. 1.4) [29], and animal studies allowed several important observations. Hossmann and colleagues [30] described the "safe revival time of the brain" as <10 min of ischemia. In 1988, they used normothermic cats to run 143 experiments of global brain ischemia of 1-h durations and noted that hyperglycemia and acidosis worsened outcome after insult [31]. Even more importantly, they observed that cats with a lower pre-ischemic temperature had improved electroencephalogram (EEG) recovery after ischemia. Safar et al. [32] also noted the advantage of "accidental" pre-ischemic hypothermia in their dog model of cardiac arrest, and this prompted their group to perform a series of five controlled experiments of ventricular

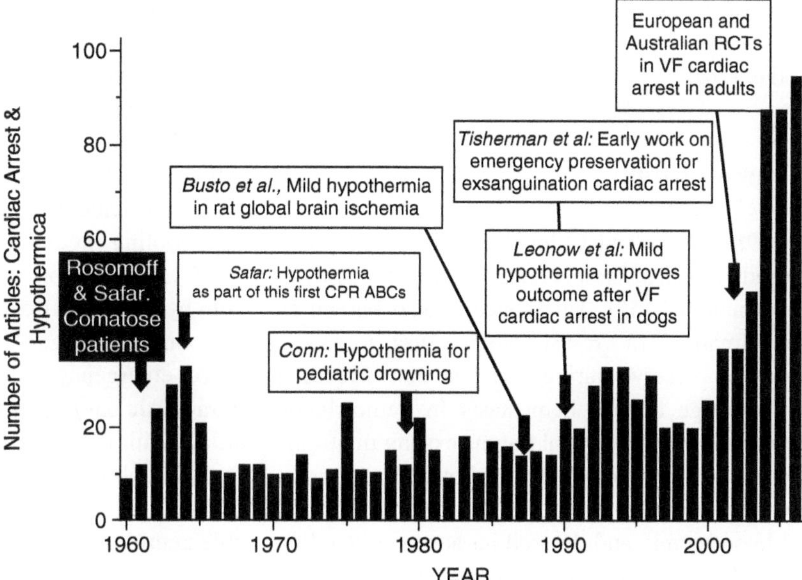

Fig. 1.4 Trend of articles on cardiac arrest & hypothermia since 1960 [29]

fibrillation in dogs [33, 34]. Varying the ischemic time and the hypothermia duration, induced within 15 min of reperfusion, the critical observation that mild hypothermia seemed to confer benefit [35], without the risks involved with moderate hypothermia, revived the study of resuscitative hypothermia for improved neurological outcome after cardiac arrest.

Independently and simultaneously, other researchers drew similar conclusions about the beneficial effect of mild resuscitative hypothermia in rat forebrain ischemia models. For example, Busto et al. [36] showed that small changes in intra-ischemic brain temperature (33, 34, 36, or 39°C) significantly worsened histopathologic necrosis. In a later experiment, they added 3 h of hypothermia in the post-ischemic period and found that immediate, but not 30-min delayed, therapy reduced hippocampal CA1 injury [37]. Interestingly, Dietrich and colleagues [38] used a similar rat forebrain model to compare outcomes in three groups of post-insult rats to evaluate the efficacy of permanent protection of postischemic hypothermia over time. One group was maintained with normothermia throughout insult and recirculation; one was treated with postischemic hypothermia, achieved within 3–5 min of recirculation; and one was treated with intraischemic hypothermia but normothermia during recirculation. Their primary findings were that short-term, not long-term, protection of hippocampal CA1 neurons was observed with postischemic hypothermia and that hypothermia may increase the therapeutic window for pharmacotherapy against delayed pathophysiological events.

Numerous variations on ischemic time, delay to hypothermia treatment, and duration of hypothermia seemed to all suggest that longer durations and minimal delay to initiation of therapy were important for best immediate and long term outcome [39–42]. The idea "the earlier the better", with regard to resuscitative hypothermia, spurred incredible research efforts to design safe, minimally invasive methods to achieve target temperature as quickly as possible [43–45]. Some focused on intravenous cold saline [46–48] and some pioneered cardiopulmonary bypass [49–52] to expedite intraischemic hypothermia. All the while, scientists were gaining a better understanding of the complex, multifactorial and staged nature of the post-ischemia process, a cascade of changes that Negovsky referred to as an iatrogenic "post-resuscitation disease" in 1983 [53]. It is this ischemia-reperfusion aftermath – global hypoperfusion and subsequent hyperemia, resulting in blood–brain barrier leakage, micro foci of incomplete ischemia, and free radical reactions – that continues to draw attention today [54].

Safar's Vision

In 1984, Safar and Colonel Bellamy [39] introduced the idea of "suspended animation for delayed resuscitation" [55]. This concept, also known as "reanimation" or "resuscitology", was born as a tactic to preserve during transport and give time for damage control hemostasis in hemorrhagic shock and otherwise fatal trauma exsanguinations. Building once again on the cardiovascular surgery experience, Safar and colleagues took advantage of hypothermia and devised an aortic cold saline flush [56] method to rapidly induce suspended animation, preserve the brain, and prolong the window for definitive resuscitation. Ideally, hypothermia would be induced prior to arrival at the hospital, where emergency cardiopulmonary bypass (ECPB) could then be instituted and used to maintain or rewarm the patient as well [39].

Suspended Animation is not as futuristic as one might have thought in the 1990s. To give a few examples, current efforts to develop cardiopulmonary bypass circuits for animal models of cardiac arrest are underway [49]; in Japan, researchers routinely initiate ECPB for OOH-CA patients, refractory to initial standard resuscitation [50, 52]; and in San Diego, Emergency Medicine physicians at Sharp Memorial Hospital have implemented ECPB in a small series of patients with success [57, 58]. The synergy between hypothermia and ECPB to create suspended animation can easily be extended to sudden asphyxiation or massive pulmonary embolism with obstructive shock, sudden pump failure with cardiovascular collapse, septic shock, and even congenital heart disease. It is a paradigm that, in theory, allows for controlled recirculation and reversal of acute death. The full therapeutic potential of Safar's vision remains to be discovered and is worthy of continued exploration [29].

> *Without faith a man can do nothing; with it all things are possible.*
>
> *– Sir William Osler*

Landmark Clinical Studies

Several small, non-randomized trials of mild therapeutic hypothermia after cardiac arrest were published in the late 1990s and early 2000s. Studies by Yanagawa et al. [59], Zeiner et al. [60], and Felberg et al. [61] used primarily surface cooling methods to reach goal temperature (33°C), and all concluded feasibility and benefit with hypothermia treatment, compared to historical controls. Nagao [52] and colleagues combined emergency cardiopulmonary bypass and intra-aortic balloon pump, to accomplish resuscitation, with hypothermia therapy for about 48 h. In their cohort, the combined cardiac and cerebral resuscitation strategy resulted in 57% favorable neurological outcome.

A total of three randomized studies [62–64], and one meta-analysis [65], on the use of hypothermia after cardiac arrest have been published, and in 2002, two were published back to back in the New England Journal of Medicine (NEJM) [62, 63]. These two multi-center, randomized clinical studies prompted re-enthusiasm for resuscitation research, echoing the work of Benson et al. [26] in 1959. While neither of the NEJM studies was without limitation, including the highly selective patient populations and the inability to blind providers to the treatment group, these independent investigations brought promise for the use of mild TH to improve neurological function after resuscitation from cardiac arrest and provoked many more questions for study.

HACA

The Hypothermia After Cardiac Arrest (HACA) study group from Europe presented a feasibility study in 2000 [60]. Statistical analysis included 27 adult, witnessed, OOH-CA patients who were cooled with mild TH for at least 24 h. The use of mild TH in these patients was concluded to be safe, with no significant bleeding or cardiovascular complications.

In 2002, the HACA group reported on a prospective, randomized, multi-center clinical trial [62]. A total of 275 adult patients (at least 18 years old) with OOH-CA from nine centers in five countries had been randomized to mild TH at 32–34°C versus standard treatment. Patients were accepted who remained comatose after witnessed OOH-CA due to ventricular fibrillation or pulseless ventricular tachycardia, who had resuscitation attempted by EMS within 15 min of collapse, and who achieved ROSC in less than 60 min. The goal time to reach target temperature was within 4 h, and surface cooling was used to maintain target temperature for 24 h. Patients were then allowed to rewarm passively.

Results from the HACA trial revealed more favorable neurological outcomes and reduced mortality in the hypothermia group. A total of 55% of the hypothermia group, versus 39% of the control group, were able to live independently and work at least part-time at 6 months. The cumulative survival between the two groups, at every time point out to 6 months after admission to the hospital, was better in the hypothermia group. While sepsis was more likely to develop in the hypothermia group, the proportion of patients with complications was not statistically different between the treatment groups, and the benefits were felt to far outweigh the risks of treatment with TH.

Bernard et al.

Bernard and collaborators in Australia first published the results of a nonrandomized clinical trial in 1997 [66]. They prospectively treated 22 adult OOH-CA patients with therapeutic hypothermia for 12 h in the ICU and made outcome comparisons with 22 matched historical controls. Their results were promising, showing both a survival and an improved neurological outcome benefit in the patients treated with hypothermia.

In 2002, they reported on a prospective, randomized clinical trial conducted in four hospitals in Melbourne, Australia [63]. A total of 43 patients were treated with TH to 33°C and 34 patients were treated with normothermia (37°C). Patients were accepted who remained comatose after OOH-CA due to ventricular fibrillation, who were males, at least 18 years of age, or females, at least 50 years of age, and were transported initially to a participating center. Surface cooling with ice packs was used to induce and then maintain target temperature for 12 h after hospital admission. Patients were actively rewarmed, starting at 18 h after admission.

Of the patients treated with TH, 49% had good neurological function at discharge. In contrast, 26% of the normothermia group had favorable neurological outcome. Importantly, both of their studies suggested the safety of mild therapeutic hypothermia treatment after OOH-CA. While hyperglycemia, hyperkalemia, decreased heart rate, and increased systemic vascular resistance were observed, there were no clinically significant adverse outcomes between the two groups.

Unanswered Questions

Treatment Targets

For the last decade (2002–present, 2012), there has not been another clinical, randomized controlled trial investigating the use of resuscitative hypothermia to improve neurological outcome after cardiac arrest. Many questions remain unanswered, such as the optimal depth and duration for therapy. In 2005, the AHA and ILCOR [54] recommended therapeutic hypothermia after cardiac arrest for 12–24 h at 32–34°C; however, experts are not entirely sure whether one-size fits-all for post-resuscitation care. The benefit of TH does consistently seem to outweigh the risk [62, 63], so these scientific bodies have urged TH to be implemented in the post-cardiac arrest bundle as standard of care.

Questions also remain regarding the optimal timing and rate of hypothermia initiation and rewarming for maximal benefit. Figure 1.5 demonstrates the temperature trends from the HACA trial for the hypothermia and control groups. Varying the timing and rate of achieving therapeutic targets will alter the relationships of these curves. Some animals studies have shown that intra-ischemic, compared to post-ischemic, initiation of hypothermia confers benefit [43, 45], while others have suggested the therapeutic window might be more variable. Animal studies have been utilized to investigate the variable time to

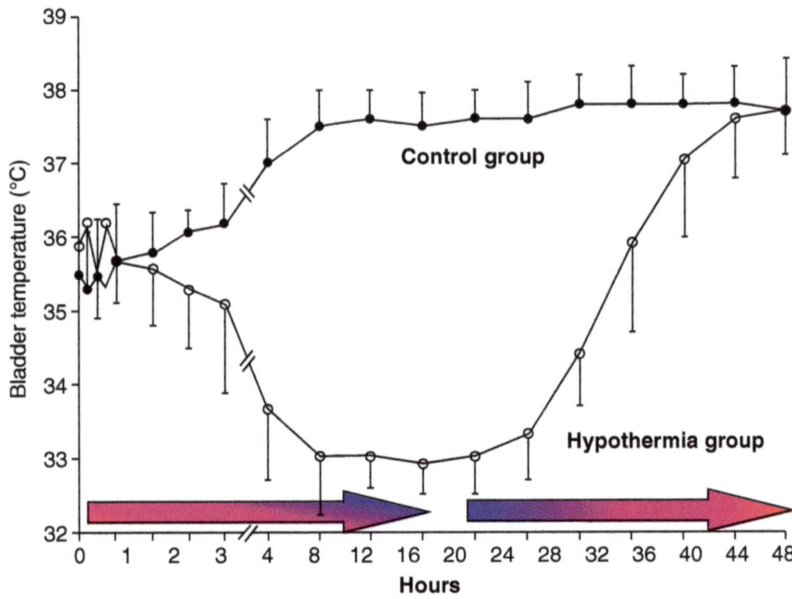

Fig. 1.5 HACA trial: bladder temperature trends, hours after ROSC [62]

target temperature, or rate at which body temperature is cooled to goal. Results again have been controversial, with some research showing that faster is better [50, 67] while others, including some human, clinical studies, have suggested that a quicker time to target temperature is associated with poorer outcome [68, 69]. Large, prospective studies are needed to gain a better understanding of when and how hypothermia is of most benefit for patients suffering from cardiopulmonary arrest.

Molecular Considerations

In 2002, Weisfeldt and Becker [70] described the three-phase model of resuscitation, based on time-sensitive physiologic pathology and suggesting specific treatment interventions depending on phase. The electrical phase extends from time of arrest to about 4 min, during which internal or external defibrillators or AEDs are most effective. The circulatory phase ranges from about 4 to 10 min after arrest. In theory, immediate defibrillation during this time might be detrimental because of the metabolic byproduct buildup resulting from ischemia. In some studies, providing 1–3 min of circulation (i.e. external CPR) allowed for improved defibrillation success. The metabolic phase, after approximately 10 min of arrest, signifies prolonged tissue injury from hypoperfusion and success from CPR and defibrillation begins to decrease. Furthermore, the risk of attaining reperfusion also increases in the metabolic phase and can result in recirculation injury. In practice, it is difficult to determine in which phase of cardiac arrest patients are found, and even if witnessed, there could be individual variability with respect to duration in each phase, due to underlying comorbidity. It is in the metabolic phase that suspended animation therapy has great potential.

In 2010, the AHA expanded the recommendation for the use of therapeutic hypothermia after cardiac arrest to be considered in the treatment of any patient after cardiac arrest with any presenting rhythm, including patients who arrest while in-hospital [71]. Further research into the ischemia-reperfusion milieu, in search of a more specific treatment target than mere core body temperature, perhaps at the immuno-metabolic level, is underway. Scientists have been investigating cellular targets, such as mitochondria, to mitigate the global reperfusion injury after cardiac arrest. While some experts postulate that therapeutic hypothermia may allow for treatment synergy, increasing the therapeutic window for pharmacologic modulators of the inflammatory cascade, others are exploring pathways to support a dose–response relationship for hypothermia. To these ends, consortia of clinical efforts have been developed, including the Resuscitation Outcomes Consortium (ROC) [72], in order to garner data from multiple treatment sites and tackle these difficult questions.

> *Faith has to do with things that are not seen and hope with things that are not at hand.*
>
> *– Thomas Aquinas*

Conclusions

The history of therapeutic hypothermia to improve neurological outcomes after cardiac arrest has only just begun. Over the last 10–15 years, researchers have taken a second look at the cardiac surgery experience, rediscovered the early work of Safar, and breathed new life into resuscitology. The recognition that organisms who survive resuscitation from acute death are subject to a complex cascade of ischemia-reperfusion injury has led to the recommendation that mild therapeutic hypothermia be part of the comprehensive post-resuscitation care bundle [73].

In time, I suspect more individualized research will be translated from bench to bedside, and as a researcher, I am eager to contribute answers to the many questions awaiting explanation. In fact, at ReSS 2011, I was given the opportunity to present the research I had completed during my fellowship, earning one of the four Best Abstract Awards. Professionally this was a huge honor; personally, I stood before my colleagues to remind them why we do what we do. As a representative survivor, I exemplify an effective chain of survival and serve to both inspire and give hope to the ongoing resurgence in resuscitation research. May the chapters that follow guide your efforts to impact outcomes after cardiac arrest, in your practice and your community.

References

1. Kouwenhoven WB, Jude JR, Knickerbocker GG. Closed-chest cardiac massage. JAMA. 1960;173:1064–7.
2. Beck CS, Leighninger DS. Death after a clean bill of health. So-called "fatal" heart attacks and treatment with resuscitation techniques. JAMA. 1960;174:133–5.
3. Safar P. Life in the balance: emergency medicine and the quest to reverse sudden death. N Engl J Med. 1997;337(3):206–7.
4. Centers for Disease Control. Morbidity and mortality weekly report; 1999;48(50):1141–7.
5. Murphy SL. Deaths: preliminary data for 2010: National vital statistics reports; 2012.
6. Sondik EJ. National Center for Health Statistics, celebrating 50 years. 2012. Available at: http://www.cdc.gov/nchs/about/50th_anniversary.htm. Accessed 6 Feb 2012.
7. Roger VL, Go AS, Lloyd-Jones DM, Benjamin EJ, Berry JD, Borden WB, Bravata DM, Dai S, Ford ES, Fox CS, Fullerton HJ, Gillespie C, Hailpern SM, Heit JA, Howard VJ, Kissela BM, Kittner SJ, Lackland DT, Lichtman JH, Lisabeth LD, Makuc DM, Marcus GM, Marelli A, Matchar DB, Moy CS, Mozaffarian D, Mussolino ME, Nichol G, Paynter NP, Soliman EZ, Sorlie PD, Sotoodehnia N, Turan TN, Virani SS, Wong ND, Woo D, Turner MB. Heart disease and stroke statistics–2012 update: a report from the American Heart Association. Circulation. 2012;125(1):e2–220.
8. Ornato JP, Becker LB, Weisfeldt ML, Wright BA. Cardiac arrest and resuscitation: an opportunity to align research prioritization and public health need. Circulation. 2010;122(18):1876–9.
9. Organization WH. Data & statistics. 2012. Available at: http://www.who.int/research/en/. Accessed 6 Feb 2012.
10. Merchant RM, Yang L, Becker LB, Berg RA, Nadkarni V, Nichol G, Carr BG, Mitra N, Bradley SM, Abella BS, Groeneveld PW. Incidence of treated cardiac arrest in hospitalized patients in the United States. Crit Care Med. 2011;39(11):2401–6.
11. Smith GB. In-hospital cardiac arrest: is it time for an in-hospital 'chain of prevention'? Resuscitation. 2010;81(9):1209–11.
12. DeVita MA, Smith GB, Adam SK, Adams-Pizarro I, Buist M, Bellomo R, Bonello R, Cerchiari E, Farlow B, Goldsmith D, Haskell H, Hillman K, Howell M, Hravnak M, Hunt EA, Hvarfner A, Kellett J, Lighthall GK, Lippert A, Lippert FK, Mahroof R, Myers JS, Rosen M, Reynolds S, Rotondi A, Rubulotta F, Winters B. "Identifying the hospitalised patient in crisis"—a consensus conference on the afferent limb of rapid response systems. Resuscitation. 2010;81(4):375–82.
13. Sayre MR, Berg RA, Cave DM, Page RL, Potts J, White RD. Hands-only (compression-only) cardiopulmonary resuscitation: a call to action for

bystander response to adults who experience out-of-hospital sudden cardiac arrest: a science advisory for the public from the American Heart Association Emergency Cardiovascular Care Committee. Circulation. 2008;117(16):2162–7.
14. American Heart Association CC. Chain of survival. 2012. Available at: http://www.heart.org/HEARTORG/CPRAndECC/WhatisCPR/ECCIntro/Chain-of-Survival_UCM_307516_Article.jsp. Accessed 6 Feb 2012.
15. Fay T. Early experiences with local and generalized refrigeration of the human brain. J Neurosurg. 1959;16(3):239–59. discussion 259–260.
16. Varon J, Acosta P. Therapeutic hypothermia: past, present, and future. Chest. 2008;133(5):1267–74.
17. Varon J, Marik PE, Einav S. Therapeutic hypothermia: a state-of-the-art emergency medicine perspective. Am J Emerg Med. 2011.
18. Botterell EH, Lougheed WM, Scott JW, Vandewater SL. Hypothermia, and interruption of carotid, or carotid and vertebral circulation, in the surgical management of intracranial aneurysms. J Neurosurg. 1956;13(1):1–42.
19. Bigelow WG, Lindsay WK, Greenwood WF. Hypothermia; its possible role in cardiac surgery: an investigation of factors governing survival in dogs at low body temperatures. Ann Surg. 1950;132(5):849–66.
20. Bigelow WG, McBirnie JE. Further experiences with hypothermia for intracardiac surgery in monkeys and groundhogs. Ann Surg. 1953;137(3):361–5.
21. Baffes TG. Hypothermia in cardiovascular surgery. J Natl Med Assoc. 1958;50(6):426–8.
22. Rosomoff HL, Holaday DA. Cerebral blood flow and cerebral oxygen consumption during hypothermia. Am J Physiol. 1954;179(1):85–8.
23. Rosomoff HL, Gilbert R. Brain volume and cerebrospinal fluid pressure during hypothermia. Am J Physiol. 1955;183(1):19–22.
24. Zimmerman JM, Spencer FC. The influence of hypothermia on cerebral injury resulting from circulatory occlusion. Surg Forum. 1958;9:216–8.
25. Williams Jr GR, Spencer FC. The clinical use of hypothermia following cardiac arrest. Ann Surg. 1958;148(3):462–8.
26. Benson DW, Williams Jr GR, Spencer FC, Yates AJ. The use of hypothermia after cardiac arrest. Anesth Analg. 1959;38:423–8.
27. Marion DW, Leonov Y, Ginsberg M, Katz LM, Kochanek PM, Lechleuthner A, Nemoto EM, Obrist W, Safar P, Sterz F, Tisherman SA, White RJ, Xiao F, Zar H. Resuscitative hypothermia. Crit Care Med. 1996;24(2 Suppl):S81–9.
28. Acierno LJ, Worrell LT. Peter Safar: father of modern cardiopulmonary resuscitation. Clin Cardiol. 2007;30(1):52–4.
29. Kochanek PM, Drabek T, Tisherman SA. Therapeutic hypothermia: the Safar vision. J Neurotrauma. 2009;26(3):417–20.
30. Hossmann KA. Post-ischemic resuscitation of the brain: selective vulnerability versus global resistance. Prog Brain Res. 1985;63:3–17.
31. Hossmann KA. Resuscitation potentials after prolonged global cerebral ischemia in cats. Crit Care Med. 1988;16(10):964–71.
32. Safar P. Resuscitation from clinical death: pathophysiologic limits and therapeutic potentials. Crit Care Med. 1988;16(10):923–41.
33. Leonov Y, Sterz F, Safar P, Radovsky A. Moderate hypothermia after cardiac arrest of 17 minutes in dogs. Effect on cerebral and cardiac outcome. Stroke. 1990;21(11):1600–6.
34. Sterz F, Safar P, Tisherman S, Radovsky A, Kuboyama K, Oku K. Mild hypothermic cardiopulmonary resuscitation improves outcome after prolonged cardiac arrest in dogs. Crit Care Med. 1991;19(3):379–89.
35. Leonov Y, Sterz F, Safar P, Radovsky A, Oku K, Tisherman S, Stezoski SW. Mild cerebral hypothermia during and after cardiac arrest improves neurologic outcome in dogs. J Cereb Blood Flow Metab. 1990;10(1):57–70.
36. Busto R, Dietrich WD, Globus MY, Valdes I, Scheinberg P, Ginsberg MD. Small differences in intraischemic brain temperature critically determine the extent of ischemic neuronal injury. J Cereb Blood Flow Metab. 1987;7(6):729–38.
37. Busto R, Dietrich WD, Globus MY, Ginsberg MD. Postischemic moderate hypothermia inhibits CA1 hippocampal ischemic neuronal injury. Neurosci Lett. 1989;101(3):299–304.
38. Dietrich WD, Busto R, Alonso O, Globus MY, Ginsberg MD. Intraischemic but not postischemic brain hypothermia protects chronically following global forebrain ischemia in rats. J Cereb Blood Flow Metab. 1993;13(4):541–9.
39. Tisherman S, Sterz F, editors. Therapeutic hypothermia. New York: Springer Science & Business Media, Inc; 2005.
40. Noguchi K, Matsumoto N, Shiozaki T, Tasaki O, Ogura H, Kuwagata Y, Sugimoto H, Seiyama A. Effects of timing and duration of hypothermia on survival in an experimental gerbil model of global ischaemia. Resuscitation. 2011;82(4):481–6.
41. Kuboyama K, Safar P, Radovsky A, Tisherman SA, Stezoski SW, Alexander H. Delay in cooling negates the beneficial effect of mild resuscitative cerebral hypothermia after cardiac arrest in dogs: a prospective, randomized study. Crit Care Med. 1993;21(9):1348–58.
42. Nozari A, Safar P, Stezoski SW, Wu X, Kostelnik S, Radovsky A, Tisherman S, Kochanek PM. Critical time window for intra-arrest cooling with cold saline flush in a dog model of cardiopulmonary resuscitation. Circulation. 2006;113(23):2690–6.
43. Abella BS, Zhao D, Alvarado J, Hamann K, Vanden Hoek TL, Becker LB. Intra-arrest cooling improves outcomes in a murine cardiac arrest model. Circulation. 2004;109(22):2786–91.

44. Wang H, Barbut D, Tsai MS, Sun S, Weil MH, Tang W. Intra-arrest selective brain cooling improves success of resuscitation in a porcine model of prolonged cardiac arrest. Resuscitation. 2010;81(5):617–21.
45. Zhao D, Abella BS, Beiser DG, Alvarado JP, Wang H, Hamann KJ, Hoek TL, Becker LB. Intra-arrest cooling with delayed reperfusion yields higher survival than earlier normothermic resuscitation in a mouse model of cardiac arrest. Resuscitation. 2008;77(2): 242–9.
46. Vanden Hoek TL, Kasza KE, Beiser DG, Abella BS, Franklin JE, Oras JJ, Alvarado JP, Anderson T, Son H, Wardrip CL, Zhao D, Wang H, Becker LB. Induced hypothermia by central venous infusion: saline ice slurry versus chilled saline. Crit Care Med. 2004;32(9 Suppl):S425–31.
47. Bernard S, Buist M, Monteiro O, Smith K. Induced hypothermia using large volume, ice-cold intravenous fluid in comatose survivors of out-of-hospital cardiac arrest: a preliminary report. Resuscitation. 2003; 56(1):9–13.
48. Kim F, Olsufka M, Carlbom D, Deem S, Longstreth Jr WT, Hanrahan M, Maynard C, Copass MK, Cobb LA. Pilot study of rapid infusion of 2 L of 4 degrees C normal saline for induction of mild hypothermia in hospitalized, comatose survivors of out-of-hospital cardiac arrest. Circulation. 2005;112(5):715–9.
49. Han F, Boller M, Guo W, Merchant RM, Lampe JW, Smith TM, Becker LB. A rodent model of emergency cardiopulmonary bypass resuscitation with different temperatures after asphyxial cardiac arrest. Resuscitation. 2010;81(1):93–9.
50. Nagao K, Kikushima K, Watanabe K, Tachibana E, Tominaga Y, Tada K, Ishii M, Chiba N, Kasai A, Soga T, Matsuzaki M, Nishikawa K, Tateda Y, Ikeda H, Yagi T. Early induction of hypothermia during cardiac arrest improves neurological outcomes in patients with out-of-hospital cardiac arrest who undergo emergency cardiopulmonary bypass and percutaneous coronary intervention. Circ J. 2010;74(1):77–85.
51. Tanimoto H, Ichinose K, Okamoto T, Yoshitake A, Tashiro M, Sakanashi Y, Ao H, Terasaki H. Rapidly induced hypothermia with extracorporeal lung and heart assist (ECLHA) improves the neurological outcome after prolonged cardiac arrest in dogs. Resuscitation. 2007;72(1):128–36.
52. Nagao K, Hayashi N, Kanmatsuse K, Arima K, Ohtsuki J, Kikushima K, Watanabe I. Cardiopulmonary cerebral resuscitation using emergency cardiopulmonary bypass, coronary reperfusion therapy and mild hypothermia in patients with cardiac arrest outside the hospital. J Am Coll Cardiol. 2000;36(3):776–83.
53. Negovsky VA, Gurvitch AM. Post-resuscitation disease–a new nosological entity. Its reality and significance. Resuscitation. 1995;30(1):23–7.
54. Nolan JP, Neumar RW, Adrie C, Aibiki M, Berg RA, Bottiger BW, Callaway C, Clark RS, Geocadin RG, Jauch EC, Kern KB, Laurent I, Longstreth WT, Merchant RM, Morley P, Morrison LJ, Nadkarni V, Peberdy MA, Rivers EP, Rodriguez-Nunez A, Sellke FW, Spaulding C, Sunde K, Hoek TV. Post-cardiac arrest syndrome: epidemiology, pathophysiology, treatment, and prognostication. A scientific statement from the International Liaison Committee on Resuscitation; the American Heart Association Emergency Cardiovascular Care Committee; the Council on Cardiovascular Surgery and Anesthesia; the Council on Cardiopulmonary, Perioperative, and Critical Care; the Council on Clinical Cardiology; the Council on Stroke. Resuscitation. 2008;79(3): 350–79.
55. Safar P, Tisherman SA, Behringer W, Capone A, Prueckner S, Radovsky A, Stezoski WS, Woods RJ. Suspended animation for delayed resuscitation from prolonged cardiac arrest that is unresuscitable by standard cardiopulmonary-cerebral resuscitation. Crit Care Med. 2000;28(11 Suppl):N214–8.
56. Behringer W, Prueckner S, Safar P, Radovsky A, Kentner R, Stezoski SW, Henchir J, Tisherman SA. Rapid induction of mild cerebral hypothermia by cold aortic flush achieves normal recovery in a dog outcome model with 20-minute exsanguination cardiac arrest. Acad Emerg Med. 2000;7(12):1341–8.
57. Dembitsky WP, Moreno-Cabral RJ, Adamson RM, Daily PO. Emergency resuscitation using portable extracorporeal membrane oxygenation. Ann Thorac Surg. 1993;55(1):304–9.
58. Shinar Z, Bellezzo J. Emergency physician initiated ECMO: our experience, Sharp Memorial Hospital, San Diego. Paper presented at: resuscitation science symposium. Orlando; 2011.
59. Yanagawa Y, Ishihara S, Norio H, Takino M, Kawakami M, Takasu A, Okamoto K, Kaneko N, Terai C, Okada Y. Preliminary clinical outcome study of mild resuscitative hypothermia after out-of-hospital cardiopulmonary arrest. Resuscitation. 1998;39(1–2): 61–6.
60. Zeiner A, Holzer M, Sterz F, Behringer W, Schorkhuber W, Mullner M, Frass M, Siostrzonek P, Ratheiser K, Kaff A, Laggner AN. Mild resuscitative hypothermia to improve neurological outcome after cardiac arrest. A clinical feasibility trial. Hypothermia After Cardiac Arrest (HACA) Study Group. Stroke. 2000;31(1): 86–94.
61. Felberg RA, Krieger DW, Chuang R, Persse DE, Burgin WS, Hickenbottom SL, Morgenstern LB, Rosales O, Grotta JC. Hypothermia after cardiac arrest: feasibility and safety of an external cooling protocol. Circulation. 2001;104(15):1799–804.
62. Hypothermia after Cardiac Arrest Study G. Mild therapeutic hypothermia to improve the neurologic outcome after cardiac arrest. N Engl J Med. 2002;346(8):549–56.
63. Bernard SA, Gray TW, Buist MD, Jones BM, Silvester W, Gutteridge G, Smith K. Treatment of comatose survivors of out-of-hospital cardiac arrest with induced hypothermia. N Engl J Med. 2002; 346(8):557–63.

64. Hachimi-Idrissi S, Corne L, Ebinger G, Michotte Y, Huyghens L. Mild hypothermia induced by a helmet device: a clinical feasibility study. Resuscitation. 2001;51(3):275–81.
65. Holzer M, Bernard SA, Hachimi-Idrissi S, Roine RO, Sterz F, Mullner M, Collaborative Group on Induced Hypothermia for Neuroprotection After Cardiac A. Hypothermia for neuroprotection after cardiac arrest: systematic review and individual patient data meta-analysis. Crit Care Med. 2005;33(2):414–8.
66. Bernard SA, Jones BM, Horne MK. Clinical trial of induced hypothermia in comatose survivors of out-of-hospital cardiac arrest. Ann Emerg Med. 1997;30(2):1 46–53.
67. Wolff B, Machill K, Schumacher D, Schulzki I, Werner D. Early achievement of mild therapeutic hypothermia and the neurologic outcome after cardiac arrest. Int J Cardiol. 2009;133(2):223–8.
68. Haugk M, Testori C, Sterz F, Uranitsch M, Holzer M, Behringer W, Herkner H, Time to Target Temperature Study G. Relationship between time to target temperature and outcome in patients treated with therapeutic hypothermia after cardiac arrest. Crit Care. 2011; 15(2):R101.
69. Vanston VJ, Lawhon-Triano M, Getts R, Prior J, Smego Jr RA. Predictors of poor neurologic outcome in patients undergoing therapeutic hypothermia after cardiac arrest. South Med J. 2010;103(4): 301–6.
70. Weisfeldt ML, Becker LB. Resuscitation after cardiac arrest: a 3-phase time-sensitive model. JAMA. 2002;288(23):3035–8.
71. Peberdy MA, Callaway CW, Neumar RW, Geocadin RG, Zimmerman JL, Donnino M, Gabrielli A, Silvers SM, Zaritsky AL, Merchant R, Vanden Hoek TL, Kronick SL. Part 9: post-cardiac arrest care: 2010 American Heart Association Guidelines for Cardiopulmonary Resuscitation and Emergency Cardiovascular Care. Circulation. 2010;122(18 Suppl 3):S768–86.
72. Consortium RO. NHLBI announces formation and funding of ROC. 2012. Available at: https://roc.uwctc.org/tiki/roc-public-home. Accessed 6 Feb 2012.
73. Sunde K, Pytte M, Jacobsen D, Mangschau A, Jensen LP, Smedsrud C, Draegni T, Steen PA. Implementation of a standardised treatment protocol for post resuscitation care after out-of-hospital cardiac arrest. Resuscitation. 2007;73(1):29–39.

2 Pre-hospital Therapeutic Hypothermia

Sarah K. Wallace and Benjamin S. Abella

Introduction

Mild therapeutic hypothermia (TH) maintained at 32–34°C for 12–24 h has been shown in clinical trials to significantly improve neurological outcomes for patients recovering from out-of-hospital cardiac arrest (OHCA), as reviewed elsewhere in this book [1, 2]. Though guidelines now recommend cooling for all patients who remain comatose after resuscitation from ventricular fibrillation OHCA, the optimal time to initiate a cooling protocol has not been specified. The question of whether it is advantageous and safe for emergency medical services (EMS) personnel to begin TH immediately post-resuscitation in the pre-hospital setting remains controversial [3]. This chapter will review the evidence on pre-hospital TH and propose an operational guide for program development among interested EMS agencies.

S.K. Wallace
Department of Emergency Medicine,
Center for Resuscitation Science, Hospital of the University of Pennsylvania, Philadelphia, PA, USA

Johns Hopkins University School of Medicine,
Baltimore, MD, USA
e-mail: swallace@jhmi.edu

B.S. Abella, M.D. MPhil (✉)
Department of Emergency Medicine,
Center for Resuscitation Science, University of Pennsylvania, 3400 Spruce Street, Ground Ravdin,
Philadelphia, PA 19104, USA
e-mail: benjamin.abella@uphs.upenn.edu

Review of the Literature

Several laboratory investigations have suggested that earlier cooling may maximize the neuroprotective benefit of TH in cardiac arrest patients, while delays in induction of the therapy may lead to worsened outcomes [4–6]. Meanwhile, a number of observational studies in humans have demonstrated the feasibility and safety of various pre-hospital cooling methods, including chilled saline infusions and surface cooling pads [7–14]. Their effect on clinically relevant outcomes is difficult to determine, given that most of the studies are small (including less than 40 patients) and lack concurrent control groups. Mooney et al. [15] reporting on a novel TH program in Minneapolis noted that that risk of death increased by 20% (95% CI, 4–39%) for every hour in which cooling was delayed. However, the authors did not observe a significant difference in survival to hospital discharge between patients who received pre-hospital cooling (defined as any type of cooling initiated before hospital arrival) and those who did not (OR = 1.36, 0.69–2.67). Their findings suggest earlier cooling may be important, but the incremental benefit of initiating TH in the pre-hospital setting requires further investigation.

Randomized clinical trials of pre-hospital TH have established that the therapy does reduce time to goal temperature compared to standard hospital-based TH. Whether this makes a clinically significant difference for patients is less clear. Kim et al. [16] found that OHCA patients cooled in the pre-hospital setting had a

J.B. Lundbye (ed.), *Therapeutic Hypothermia After Cardiac Arrest*,
DOI 10.1007/978-1-4471-2951-6_2, © Springer-Verlag London 2012

Table 2.1 Summary of key components of a pre-hospital TH protocol

Components	Options
Induction method	30 mL/kg intravenous ice cold saline to max 2 L
	Surface cooling (ice packs or cooling pads)
	Combination of both
Temperature measurement	Tympanic
	Esophageal
	Rectal
	Bladder
Training and education	Of EMS providers
	Of hospital personnel
	Of lay public
	Maintenance training
Quality assurance	Core temperature upon initiation of cooling
	Core temperature upon hospital arrival
	Volume of fluid delivered (if over 2 L, justify)
	Follow up with hospitals to determine if TH continued (if not, why)
System considerations	Transport times
	Hospital experience in TH and speed at initiation
	Tiered system whereby first responders can provide cooling equipment

significantly lower core body temperature upon emergency department arrival (34.7 ± 1.2°C) than a control group (35.7 ± 1.2°C) ($p<0.0001$). The authors also observed a trend towards improved survival in patients with a presenting rhythm of ventricular fibrillation (VF). Among patients cooled by pre-hospital personnel, 19/29 (66%) survived to hospital discharge, while among controls cooled in the hospital, 10/22 survived (45%). However, this difference was not statistically significant.

In another clinical trial, Bernard et al. [17] randomized 234 patients with a diagnosis of VF OHCA to either pre-hospital cooling or standard cooling after hospital admission. The authors observed a significant decrease in core body temperature upon emergency department arrival among the pre-hospital group (34.4 ± 1.2°C) compared to the standard group (35.2 ± 1.0°C) ($p<0.001$). However, they were unable to demonstrate a significant increase in 'favorable outcomes', defined as discharge home or to a rehabilitation facility; in fact, enrollment in this study was stopped early due to futility. Of note, cooling and transport were completed by an urban EMS system in Melbourne, Australia, which delivered patients quickly to hospitals with advanced experience in TH protocols. Patients in both the treatment and control arms had equivalent core temperatures at 60 min after arrival in the emergency department. Thus, the trial's findings may not be generalizable to systems with longer transport times and/or receiving hospitals less experienced with cooling.

In summary, pre-hospital TH has been shown in the literature to be safe, feasible, and effective at achieving goal temperatures more quickly than standard, hospital-based TH. However, the clinical benefit of the therapy may be greater for EMS systems with longer transport times, or those that anticipate significant delays to cooling at receiving hospitals if TH is not initiated in the field. For further exploration of the literature on pre-hospital TH, readers may seek out review articles by Leary et al. [18]. (Table 2.1) and Cabanas et al. [19].

Operational Guide

Not long ago, the practice of pre-hospital TH was rare. A 2007 survey of EMS Medical Directors and non-Medical Director EMS Physicians representing 34 US states revealed that only 6% of agencies had a protocol in place. Among these, there was wide variation in methods of cooling patients and monitoring core body temperature [20]. Today, EMS leaders are increasingly aware of the simplicity, cost effectiveness, and safety of pre-hospital cooling, despite mixed evidence in the literature regarding its clinical benefit. Among the largest US EMS systems, the majority have intentions to initiate TH protocols or are already cooling (Myers B, personal communication, 2011). Programs will soon be in development nationwide, highlighting the need for an operational, evidence-based guide for EMS leaders. The intent of this section is to familiarize readers with issues to consider and appropriate, standardized steps to take when rolling out a new pre-hospital TH program.

Inclusion Criteria

No guidelines exist outlining the inclusion criteria for pre-hospital TH. However, hospital-based TH is a class 1 indication for comatose post-arrest patients with a presenting rhythm of VF. The following minimum standards should be considered for pre-hospital cooling at this time:

1. The patient should have achieved return of spontaneous circulation (ROSC) after suffering an OHCA not related to blunt or penetrating trauma or hemorrhage;
2. The patient should have no purposeful response to pain; and
3. A receiving hospital capable of continuing TH should be identified.

Additional criteria may be added to protocols depending on the comfort level of the EMS system. These include age restrictions (e.g. >12 years with adult body habitus); temperature restrictions (core temperature after ROSC >34°C); and pregnancy restrictions (e.g. not obviously pregnant).

Induction Methods

Cold Intravenous Fluids

Patient cooling in the pre-hospital setting may be successfully achieved through rapid infusion of a large volume of ice-cold crystalloid solution. Studies have demonstrated the feasibility, safety, and efficacy of this method in inducing mild hypothermia in the field [8, 16]. Cold saline is widely considered the method of choice for pre-hospital induction of TH for its effectiveness, ease, and low cost.

However, the infusion method has several limitations. It may take up to 30 min to infuse 2 L of chilled saline, the target volume for induction of TH [8]. In one clinical trial, over half of study subjects did not receive the target 2 L due to rapid transport to the hospital before infusion was complete [17]. Thus, EMS systems with short transport times and close hospital proximity may not see as dramatic a cooling effect as systems with longer transport intervals. Conversely, rural EMS systems with extended transport times may find themselves completing infusion of 2 L chilled saline before hospital arrival. In these systems, infusion may not be an appropriate method to sustain cooling during transport, as pre-hospital infusion of greater than 2 L has not been studied in OHCA patients and may lead to volume overload. Such systems may need to add ice packs or cooling blankets to their protocol to sustain core temperatures until hospital arrival. An additional disadvantage of chilled saline is its tendency to warm towards ambient temperature during infusion. The development of insulated tubing has been proposed as a solution [21].

Despite these limitations, chilled saline remains a simple, inexpensive, and effective means of inducing hypothermia in the field for the majority of EMS agencies in the United States (Fig. 2.1).

Surface Cooling

Non-invasive whole body surface cooling with pads has been shown to be safe and feasible in the pre-hospital setting [12] (Fig. 2.2a). However, this method may afford less rapid induction than infused saline; in one study, the median time to a target temperature of 33°C was 70 (55–106) min [12]. Ice packs or cooling pads may play an important supplementary role to chilled saline methods, both before infusion to expedite cooling and after infusion to maintain target temperature (Fig. 2.2b).

Temperature Measurement

Overcooling in the pre-hospital setting below 32°C can increase a patient's risk for arrhythmia and coagulopathy. One retrospective study of TH at three hospitals noted that unintentional overcooling was common, even in the induction phase. This was especially true when simple cooling methods such as IV fluids and ice packs were used without thermostatic monitoring [22]. It is therefore important that EMS personnel have access to accurate

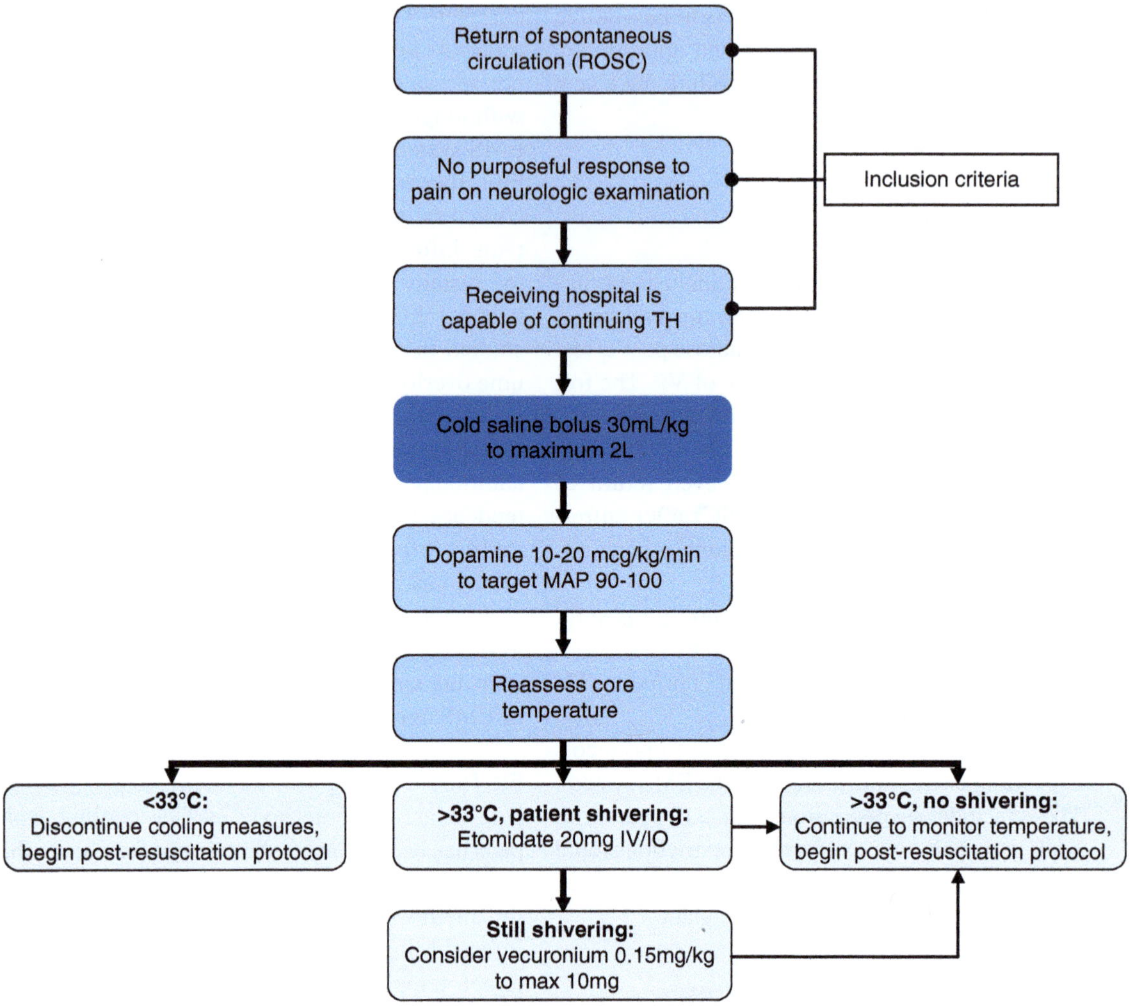

Return of spontaneous circulation (ROSC)

No purposeful response to pain on neurologic examination

Receiving hospital is capable of continuing TH

Inclusion criteria

Cold saline bolus 30mL/kg to maximum 2L

Dopamine 10-20 mcg/kg/min to target MAP 90-100

Reassess core temperature

<33°C: Discontinue cooling measures, begin post-resuscitation protocol

>33°C, patient shivering: Etomidate 20mg IV/IO

>33°C, no shivering: Continue to monitor temperature, begin post-resuscitation protocol

Still shivering: Consider vecuronium 0.15mg/kg to max 10mg

Fig. 2.1 Example pre-hospital TH protocol (Adapted from Wake County EMS Induced Hypothermia Protocol, available at http://www.wakeems.com/ICE/ihv11.13.pdf)

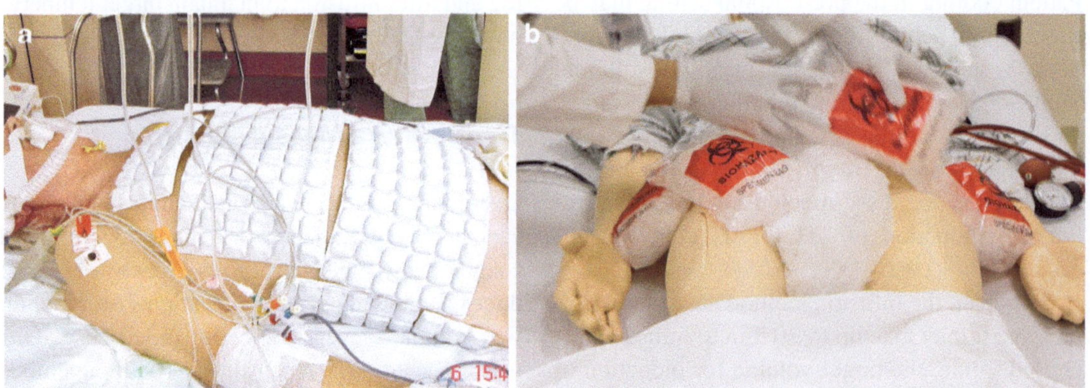

Fig. 2.2 Pre-hospital TH induction methods. Four examples of cooling methods, shown for illustrative purposes: (**a**) Surface cooling with flexible pads (EMCOOLS; Vienna, Austria). (**b**) Surface cooling with ice packs (U.S. photo/Staff Sgt. Keyonna Fennell). (**c**) Trans-nasal evaporative cooling (BeneChill; Lausanne, Switzerland). (**d**) Intravenous cooling with chilled saline

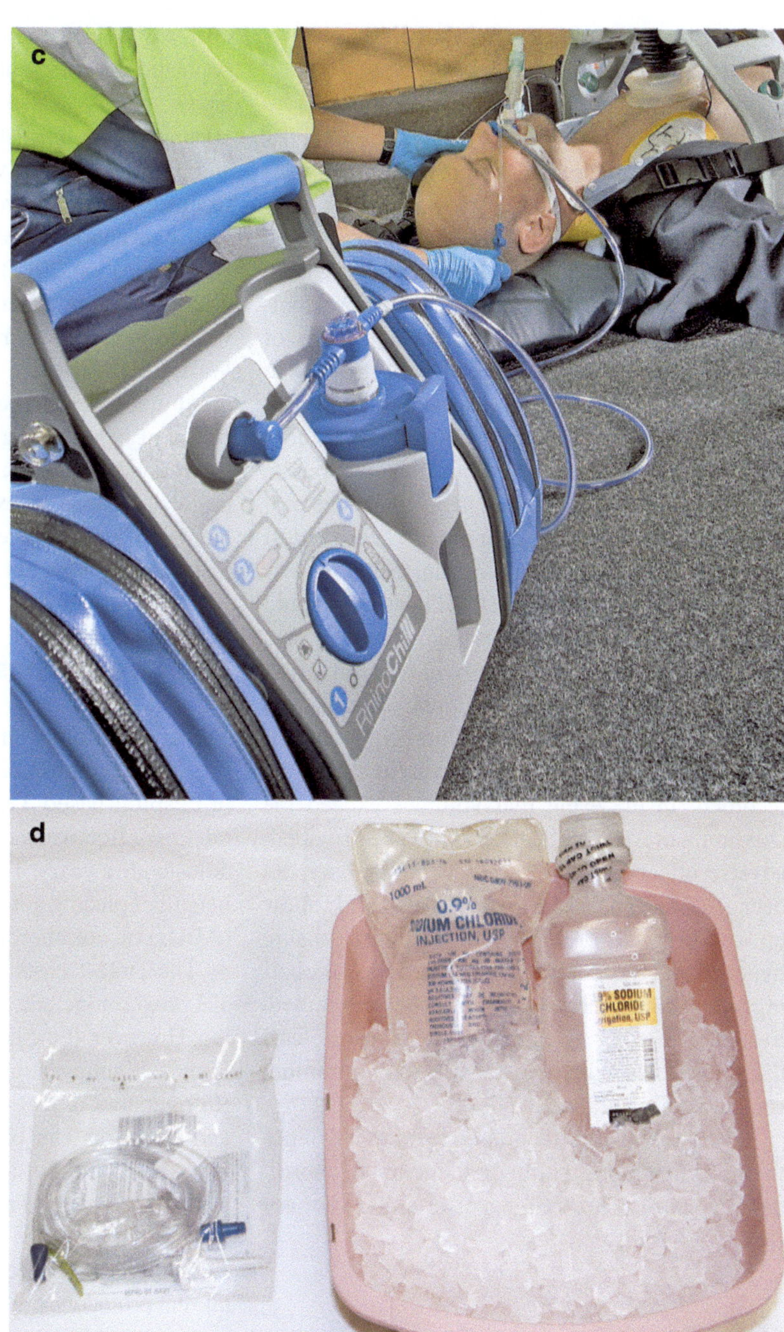

Fig. 2.2 (continued)

methods for temperature monitoring when inducing TH in the pre-hospital setting.

Tympanic thermometer devices are generally inexpensive, readily available, and easily and rapidly usable. Tympanic temperature measurement may be less reliable than other methods of temperature measurement, such as esophageal, bladder, or rectal temperature [23]. Nevertheless, it remains a reasonable choice for use in the pre-hospital setting since other measures may be more cumbersome in practice. Upon arrival at the hospital, core temperature should be monitored using one of the more reliable measurement tools, such as bladder or esophageal probes.

Education, Training, and Quality Assurance

Education and training of EMS providers and hospital personnel are crucial steps towards the implementation of a successful pre-hospital cooling protocol. Initial education and training can be time-intensive, but maintenance training is typically minimal given the relative simplicity of cooling and its alignment with the existing skills of pre-hospital personnel. Wake County EMS in North Carolina spent 8 months training EMS providers and receiving hospital personnel on its cold saline protocol, as well as educating the public through community-wide initiatives. Since the program began, maintenance training has been modest (Myers B, personal communication, 2011).

Built into any pre-hospital TH protocol should be a means of quality assurance. Temperatures should be recorded by EMS providers upon initiation of cooling in the field and upon arrival at the hospital. If utilizing a cold saline protocol, volumes of fluid delivered to each patient should be recorded. In the event that volumes exceed the maximum of 2 L, justification should be provided; adverse effects at these larger volumes have not been studied. Finally, EMS systems should follow up with hospitals on all cooled patients to ensure hypothermia was continued after delivery. If cooling was stopped, the reason should be determined. Systemic monitoring and evaluation of at least these variables will help ensure that minimum standards of quality are achieved.

EMS leaders are encouraged to cultivate hypothermia champions within their agency to coordinate education and training efforts and monitor quality assurance.

EMS Systems Considerations

EMS response system characteristics may be exploited to provide access to cooling equipment for pre-hospital personnel while streamlining cost and training. For example, EMS agencies with a tiered system could spare the majority of providers from the burden of training and time: firefighters or EMT-certified first responders with cooling equipment could coordinate with standard EMS to respond to OHCAs. Wake County EMS, a system that serves a population of one million and includes 50 ambulances, has dedicated ten vehicles to pre-hospital cooling and equipped them with electric refrigerators and cold saline. These vehicles respond to OHCAs to facilitate the administration of cold fluids in parallel with conventional EMS care (Myers B, personal communication, 2011). Such a protocol is cost effective, reliable, and potentially life saving; overall survival from OHCA increased from 8.1% to 11.5% in Wake County in the year following initiation of their pre-hospital TH program, though the relative contribution of field cooling to this increase could not be determined due to lack of a control group [14]. If this protocol were to be exported to other systems, the number of equipped vehicles may be adjusted based on an agency's patient volume and area covered.

Cost Effectiveness

There are no published cost-benefit analyses specific to pre-hospital TH at present. In one study of hospital-based TH, cooling had an incremental cost-effectiveness ratio of $100,000/quality adjusted life years. This is comparable to the cost-benefit of placing automated external defibrillators (AEDs) on commercial US airlines [24].

The largest costs of developing a pre-hospital TH program include equipment, storage, and training. However, if the chosen method of inducing TH is via cold intravenous fluids, costs can be minimal. Refrigerators or readily available beverage coolers and ice packs can be placed in EMS vehicles to keep fluids cold. Little education on the part of pre-hospital personnel is required as infusion of saline is well within the scope of their duties. Newer cooling technologies may increase cost barriers, but under current protocols, pre-hospital TH is relatively inexpensive even for resource-poor agencies.

Logistical Concerns

EMS systems often operate under conditions of limited resources and staffing. The development of a pre-hospital TH program could conceivably increase the workload of EMS providers and potentially interrupt other post-arrest patient care priorities such as airway management and swift transport to the hospital. According to a 2007 survey, barriers to cooling among EMS agencies included overburden with other tasks, lack of refrigeration capabilities, short transport times, and the perception that receiving hospitals would not continue hypothermia efforts. Lack of specific guidelines and scientific consensus regarding the use of pre-hospital cooling were also identified as obstacles [20]. These concerns highlight the complexity of developing an effective algorithm for pre-hospital TH programs and should be addressed by EMS directors wishing to develop protocols for cooling.

The individual characteristics of a given EMS system should be taken into consideration when weighing the incremental benefit of pre-hospital cooling against its costs in terms of time and resources. For example, in systems featuring reasonably short transport times (less than 10 min) and the ability to deliver patients to TH-experienced receiving hospitals where hypothermia is initiated within an hour of arrival, field cooling may not be justified. However, EMS agencies with longer transport times and/or a tiered response system whereby first responders could share the cost and responsibility of cooling protocols, the development of a pre-hospital TH program may be more appropriate. Moreover, it has been suggested that in communities where receiving hospitals are slow or hesitant to perform standard TH, initiation of cooling in the field may encourage continuation of hypothermia by hospitals. In this way, despite mixed evidence on its direct benefit, pre-hospital cooling may have an indirect effect on survival and neurological outcome by forcing the hand of hospital providers to provide prompt, sustained hypothermia in resuscitated patients.

Adverse Events

Documented adverse events from published trials of pre-hospital TH have been modest and likely of small clinical consequence [7–10, 12, 13, 16, 17, 25]. However, the potential still exists for arrhythmias, electrolyte disorders, infection, bleeding, and seizures [26]. Shivering increases oxygen consumption and leads to warming, impeding the induction of hypothermia; therefore, it should be prevented by administration of sedation and a neuromuscular blockade such as etomidate or vecuronium [27]. Of note, shivering is rare in the pre-hospital setting, with less than 5% of cases requiring neuromuscular blockade, although additional work is required to document shivering incidence in the pre-hospital environment [18]. (Myers B, personal communication, 2011). Cold saline is a potential vasoconstrictor, so mean arterial pressure (MAP) should be monitored closely. If chilled saline does not maintain MAP to a target level of approximately 80 mm Hg or greater, vasopressor agents should be considered. Patients may develop metabolic alkalosis with cooling, so hyperventilation should be avoided.

Guidelines for the prevention and treatment of common adverse events such as these should be outlined in pre-hospital TH protocols so that providers can predict and manage them effectively.

Future Directions

Pre-hospital TH is an area ripe for investigation. Many new studies have been proposed to investigate alternative induction methods, the optimal timing of cooling, and more. Providers should be aware of the following future directions for pre-hospital TH research.

Alternative Induction Methods

Trans-nasal Evaporative Cooling

Trans-nasal evaporative cooling is one promising new technology under evaluation for pre-hospital TH induction. A clinical trial by Castren et al. [28] demonstrated the safety, feasibility, and efficacy of this method using a delivery device called the RhinoChill. This device sprays a liquid coolant-oxygen mixture into the nasal cavity of OHCA patients with subsequent evaporation by virtue of high-flow oxygen. The RhinoChill is designed as a portable device and can be set up for emergent use within minutes. The authors found a non-significant trend towards increased survival among trans-nasally cooled patients compared to controls (43.8% versus 31.0%, $p=0.26$), and a significant difference in survival among a subset of patients who had CPR initiated within 10 min of collapse (56.5% in the nasally cooled group versus 29.4% among controls, p=0.04). Although not yet FDA-approved for use on OHCA patients in the United States, trans-nasal cooling devices such as the RhinoChill are on the horizon for pre-hospital TH induction (Fig. 2.2c).

Saline/Ice Slurries

Laboratory studies have suggested that intravenous infusion of micro-particulate ice slurries may be another means of rapid induction of TH in the pre-hospital setting. One study in swine demonstrated that ice slurry cooled more rapidly than an equal volume of chilled saline after central catheter infusion [29]. However, the use of slurries in humans has not been studied.

Chilled Perfluorocarbons

Ventilation with perfluorocarbons (PFCs) – inert liquids with oxygen carrying properties – is another novel technique under laboratory investigation for induction of TH. This method has the potential to rapidly cool the pulmonary vascular bed. Laboratory studies have found that liquid ventilation with cold PFCs can induce TH rapidly and without adverse effects [30], and may even increase the rate of ROSC compared to chilled saline when administered in the intra-arrest period [31].

Timing

Researchers have postulated that initiating TH <u>during</u> resuscitation efforts instead of <u>after</u> return of spontaneous circulation (ROSC) might maximize the therapy's benefit, or perhaps even exert an independent effect on clinical recovery. In one retrospective study of 551 patients, Garrett et al. [32] documented an improved rate of pre-hospital ROSC after infusion of cold saline during the intra-arrest period (OR 1.83; 95% CI 1.19–2.81). The authors also observed a trend towards increased survival to hospital admission and discharge among patients receiving intra-arrest TH; however, these findings did not reach statistical significance. TH initiated during resuscitation efforts as opposed to post-ROSC could lead to earlier brain cooling and may be associated with improved outcomes. However, the feasibility and clinical efficacy of intra-arrest TH should be evaluated in a randomized, controlled trial before conclusions are drawn regarding its superiority to post-ROSC cooling.

Rhythm

In a clinical trial conducted by Kim et al. [16] pre-hospital cooling in patients with VF was associated with a trend towards improved survival to hospital discharge. However, in patients presenting with non-VF rhythms such as PEA or asystole, field cooling was associated with the reverse – a trend towards decreased survival to discharge. These findings were preliminary and not statistically significant, but merit reexamination in future studies.

Conclusions

As evidence supporting the use of hospital-based TH in the care of OHCA patients continues to mount, the appropriateness of pre-hospital TH remains unclear. Observational studies and clinical trials have suggested that pre-hospital cooling is feasible, safe, and effective at reducing core temperatures. Yet, these investigations have yet to demonstrate a difference in clinically significant outcomes. Further investigations of pre-hospital TH are needed, including those studying new methods to more rapidly induce cooling and the benefits of intra-arrest cooling.

EMS directors interested in developing a pre-hospital TH protocol should first appraise their individual EMS system and hospital capabilities. Pre-hospital TH may be more appropriate in systems that feature medium to longer response times and/or deliver to hospitals that are less timely at initiating TH. In the latter case, field initiation may have the added benefit of encouraging hospital-based cooling to avoid re-warming. In this way, pre-hospital cooling could lead to improved standard TH, a therapy with known clinical benefit. EMS systems with fast response times who deliver to TH-experienced receiving hospitals may benefit less from pre-hospital TH programs. It is at the discretion of EMS directors to determine if the benefits of pre-hospital cooling outweigh the added financial and time burdens, which fortunately are not large.

References

1. Hypothermia After Cardiac Arrest Study Group. Mild therapeutic hypothermia to improve the neurologic outcome after cardiac arrest. N Engl J Med. 2002;346(8):549–56.
2. Bernard SA, Gray TW, Buist MD, et al. Treatment of comatose survivors of out-of-hospital cardiac arrest with induced hypothermia. N Engl J Med. 2002;346(8): 557–63.
3. Emergency Cardiac Care Committee. 2005 American Heart Association Guidelines for cardiopulmonary resuscitation and emergency cardiovascular care. Circulation. 2005;112(24 Suppl):IV1–203.
4. Kuboyama K, Safar P, Radovsky A, Tisherman SA, Stezoski SW, Alexander H. Delay in cooling negates the beneficial effect of mild resuscitative cerebral hypothermia after cardiac arrest in dogs: a prospective, randomized study. Crit Care Med. 1993;21(9): 1348–58.
5. Abella BS, Zhao D, Alvarado J, Hamann K, Vanden Hoek TL, Becker LB. Intra-arrest cooling improves outcomes in a murine cardiac arrest model. Circulation. 2004;109(22):2786–91.
6. Nozari A, Safar P, Stezoski SW, et al. Critical time window for intra-arrest cooling with cold saline flush in a dog model of cardiopulmonary resuscitation. Circulation. 2006;113(23):2690–6.
7. Callaway CW, Tadler SC, Katz LM, Lipinski CL, Brader E. Feasibility of external cranial cooling during out-of-hospital cardiac arrest. Resuscitation. 2002;52(2): 159–65.
8. Virkkunen I, Yli-Hankala A, Silfvast T. Induction of therapeutic hypothermia after cardiac arrest in prehospital patients using ice-cold Ringer's solution: a pilot study. Resuscitation. 2004;62(3):299–302.
9. Kamarainen A, Virkkunen I, Tenhunen J, Yli-Hankala A, Silfvast T. Prehospital induction of therapeutic hypothermia during CPR: a pilot study. Resuscitation. 2008;76(3):360–3.
10. Storm C, Schefold JC, Kerner T, et al. Prehospital cooling with hypothermia caps (PreCoCa): a feasibility study. Clin Res Cardiol. 2008;97(10):768–72.
11. Bruel C, Parienti JJ, Marie W, et al. Mild hypothermia during advanced life support: a preliminary study in out-of-hospital cardiac arrest. Crit Care. 2008;12(1): R31.
12. Uray T, Malzer R. Out-of-hospital surface cooling to induce mild hypothermia in human cardiac arrest: a feasibility trial. Resuscitation. 2008;77(3):331–8.
13. Hammer L, Vitrat F, Savary D, et al. Immediate prehospital hypothermia protocol in comatose survivors of out-of-hospital cardiac arrest. Am J Emerg Med. 2009;27(5):570–3.
14. Hinchey PR, Myers JB, Lewis R, et al. Improved out-of-hospital cardiac arrest survival after the sequential implementation of 2005 AHA guidelines for compressions, ventilations, and induced hypothermia: the Wake County experience. Ann Emerg Med. 2010; 56(4):348–57.
15. Mooney MR, Unger BT, Boland LL, et al. Therapeutic hypothermia after out-of-hospital cardiac arrest: evaluation of a regional system to increase access to cooling. Circulation. 2011;124(2):206–14.
16. Kim F, Olsufka M, Longstreth Jr WT, et al. Pilot randomized clinical trial of prehospital induction of mild hypothermia in out-of-hospital cardiac arrest patients with a rapid infusion of 4 degrees C normal saline. Circulation. 2007;115(24):3064–70.
17. Bernard SA, Smith K, Cameron P, et al. Induction of therapeutic hypothermia by paramedics after resuscitation from out-of-hospital ventricular fibrillation cardiac arrest: a randomized controlled trial. Circulation. 2010;122(7):737–42.
18. Leary M, Vanek F, Abella BS. Prehospital use of therapeutic hypothermia after resuscitation from cardiac arrest. Ther Hypothermia Temp Manag. 2011;1(2): 69–75.
19. Cabanas JG, Brice JH, De Maio VJ, Myers B, Hinchey PR. Field-induced therapeutic hypothermia for neuroprotection after out-of hospital cardiac arrest: a systematic review of the literature. J Emerg Med. 2011;40(4):400–9.
20. Suffoletto BP, Salcido DD, Menegazzi JJ. Use of prehospital-induced hypothermia after out-of-hospital cardiac arrest: a survey of the National Association of Emergency Medical Services Physicians. Prehosp Emerg Care. 2008;12(1):52–6.
21. Mader TJ. The effect of ambient temperature on cold saline during simulated infusion to induce therapeutic hypothermia. Resuscitation. 2009;80(7):766–8.
22. Merchant RM, Abella BS, Peberdy MA, et al. Therapeutic hypothermia after cardiac arrest: unintentional overcooling is common using ice packs and conventional cooling blankets. Crit Care Med. 2006;34(12 Suppl):S490–4.
23. Moran JL, Peter JV, Solomon PJ, et al. Tympanic temperature measurements: are they reliable in the critically ill? A clinical study of measures of agreement. Crit Care Med. 2007;35(1):155–64.
24. Merchant RM, Becker LB, Abella BS, Asch DA, Groeneveld PW. Cost-effectiveness of therapeutic hypothermia after cardiac arrest. Circ Cardiovasc Qual Outcomes. 2009;2(5):421–8.
25. Kamarainen A, Virkkunen I, Tenhunen J, Yli-Hankala A, Silfvast T. Prehospital therapeutic hypothermia for comatose survivors of cardiac arrest: a randomized controlled trial. Acta Anaesthesiol Scand. 2009;53(7): 900–7.
26. Nielsen N, Sunde K, Hovdenes J, et al. Adverse events and their relation to mortality in out-of-hospital cardiac arrest patients treated with therapeutic hypothermia. Crit Care Med. 2011;39(1):57–64.
27. Nolan JP, Morley PT, Vanden Hoek TL, et al. Therapeutic hypothermia after cardiac arrest: an

advisory statement by the advanced life support task force of the International Liaison Committee on Resuscitation. Circulation. 2003;108(1):118–21.
28. Castren M, Nordberg P, Svensson L, et al. Intra-arrest transnasal evaporative cooling: a randomized, prehospital, multicenter study (PRINCE: Pre-ROSC Intra-Nasal Cooling Effectiveness). Circulation. 2010; 122(7): 729–36.
29. Vanden Hoek TL, Kasza KE, Beiser DG, et al. Induced hypothermia by central venous infusion: saline ice slurry versus chilled saline. Crit Care Med. 2004;32(9 Suppl):S425–31.
30. Staffey KS, Dendi R, Brooks LA, et al. Liquid ventilation with perfluorocarbons facilitates resumption of spontaneous circulation in a swine cardiac arrest model. Resuscitation. 2008;78(1):77–84.
31. Riter HG, Brooks LA, Pretorius AM, Ackermann LW, Kerber RE. Intra-arrest hypothermia: both cold liquid ventilation with perfluorocarbons and cold intravenous saline rapidly achieve hypothermia, but only cold liquid ventilation improves resumption of spontaneous circulation. Resuscitation. 2009;80(5): 561–6.
32. Garrett JS, Studnek JR, Blackwell T, et al. The association between intra-arrest therapeutic hypothermia and return of spontaneous circulation among individuals experiencing out of hospital cardiac arrest. Resuscitation. 2011;82(1):21–5.

Molecular Mechanism of Reperfusion Injury

3

Shoji Yokobori, M. Ross Bullock, and W. Dalton Dietrich

In the 1950s, hypothermia was induced prior to surgery to assist procedures that caused prolonged ischemia, including heart surgery [1–3] and organ transplants [4]. Within its first decade, hypothermia was applied to emergent medical situations that were characterized by cerebral ischemia and stroke [5, 6] myocardial infarction (MI) [7, 8], and cardiac arrest patients [9, 10]_ENREF_10.

The protective mechanisms of hypothermia in ischemic/reperfusion (I/R) injury are likely to be multifactorial and include both cellular and molecular events. The plausible effects of hypothermia are demonstrated especially in the early stage of the I/R injury with the best evidence to date coming from studying hypothermia in cardiac arrest patients [11, 12]. In fact, the rationale for these clinical trials mainly focused on the specific potential for therapeutic hypothermia to reduce the effects of reperfusion injury and act as a neuroprotectant.

In the field of MI, many animal studies have also demonstrated benefits of early cooling [7, 13–15]. Currently, larger human clinical trials are required to investigate the beneficial effect of hypothermia therapy on reducing myocardial infarction size and coronary reperfusion injuries [16].

To develop a deeper understanding of the benefits of therapeutic hypothermia in I/R injury, and for better comprehension of safer methodology, we reviewed and summarized several articles which help clarify the mechanisms and the efficacy of therapeutic hypothermia especially in I/R injury.

The Definition of Reperfusion Injury

During an ischemic period, the extent of tissue damage mainly relates to two major factors. One is the severity of blood flow reductions in tissue during the ischemic interval, and another is the duration of the ischemic period [17, 18]. On the return of blood flow, there is a resumption of the functions of tissue perfusion. The restored perfusion contributes to the ischemic damage process and serves to recovery of at least some of the reversibly injured tissue to a normal function. However, there is a consensus that recovery of blood flow in the post-ischemic period also has a dark side [19, 20]. Reciprocal actions between blood flow and the ischemic tissue can lead to further tissue damage. This

S. Yokobori, M.D., Ph.D.
Department of Emergency and Critical Care Medicine, Nippon Medical School, Tokyo, Japan

Department of Neurosurgery, Miami Project to Cure Paralysis, University of Miami Miller School of Medicine, Miami, FL, USA

M.R. Bullock, M.D., Ph.D. • W.D. Dietrich, Ph.D. (✉)
Department of Neurosurgery, Miami Project to Cure Paralysis, University of Miami Miller School of Medicine, Miami, FL, USA
e-mail: rbullock@med.miami.edu; ddietrich@miami.edu

J.B. Lundbye (ed.), *Therapeutic Hypothermia After Cardiac Arrest*,
DOI 10.1007/978-1-4471-2951-6_3, © Springer-Verlag London 2012

harmful aspect of return of blood perfusion has been characterized as reperfusion injury. Reperfusion damage occurs in many different types of tissues, but the majority of research has been conducted in the brain and heart.

In this regard, Ames et al. first described the potential contribution of reperfusion impairment to neural tissue damage [21]. As already noted, brain reperfusion following cerebral ischemia occurs under many kinds of clinical conditions. Transient cessation of circulation is a typical consequence during cardiac arrest and subsequent cardiopulmonary resuscitation. The breakdown or movement of emboli or clots is a common example of a transient ischemic attack and a subsequent return of normal cerebral circulation. The development of thrombolytic agents including tissue plasminogen activation (tPA) has also increased the likelihood of reperfusion after variable periods of ischemia [22].

Reperfusion injury in MI was first described by Jennings et al. [23] in their description of the histological features of the reperfused ischemic canine myocardium. This group described swelling of myocardial cells, contracture of myofibrils, disruption of the sarcolemma, and the appearance of intramitochondrial calcium phosphate particles. The reperfusion injury in myocardium is thought to involve four components of cardiac dysfunction [24]. The first is the myocardial stunning, a term defined as "mechanical dysfunction that persists after reperfusion with the absence of irreversible damage and despite restoration of normal or near-normal circulation" [25]. The myocardium usually recovers from this reversible form of injury a within several days. The second part of cardiac malfunction, the no-reflow phenomenon, was originally noted as the "inability to reperfuse a previously ischemic region" [26]. It refers to the resistance of a normal return of blood flow into the microvascular circulation encountered during opening of the infract-induced occluded coronary vessels [27]. The third of cardiac dysfunction, "reperfusion arrhythmia", is usually harmful, but effective treatments are available [28]. The last is the lethal reperfusion injury. Lethal reperfusion injury as an independent mediator of cardiomyocyte death that is distinct from ischemic injury. This concept has been debated with some researchers suggesting that reperfusion only exacerbates the cellular injury that was sustained during the ischemic period [29]. The uncertainty relates to the inability to accurately assess in situ the progress of necrosis during the transition from myocardial ischemia to reperfusion [30]. As a result, the most convincing means of showing the existence of lethal reperfusion injury as a distinct mediator of cardiomyocyte death is to show that the size of a myocardial infarct can be reduced by an intervention used at the beginning of myocardial reperfusion [30, 31].

Mechanism of Reperfusion Injury

Despite much efforts of research, the exact mechanisms of the I/R brain injury itself remain unclear. Reperfusion following ischemia can cause neurovascular injury leading to detrimental changes in blood brain barrier (BBB) permeability, cerebral edema, brain hemorrhage, and neuronal death by apoptosis/necrosis [22]. These complications clearly limit the benefits of reperfusion therapies. For example, in the clinical situation, reperfusion after brain ischemia often leads to intraparenchymal hemorrhage and severe brain swelling resulting in relatively poor outcomes.

The processes leading to brain damage after I/R injury are complex and multi-factorial. At this point the pathology of I/R injury has been separated into two distinct mechanisms. One is the cell death following cellular dysfunction, i.e., excitotoxicity, acidotoxicity and ionic imbalance. This first process is seen primarily occurring during the ischemic phase. The other type of injury comes from free radical production and oxidative stress, and this becomes particularly worst during the early reperfusion phase [32]. Together these mechanisms create a complicated picture of injury (Fig. 3.1).

In the ischemic phase, brain ischemia initiates a cascade of destructive and often irreversible processes that destroy brain cells and tissue. One example of this is the intracellular conversion to anaerobic metabolism [33]. Depletion of adenosine triphosphate (ATP) in the absence of oxidative metabolism leads to failure of the Na^+/K^+ ATPase

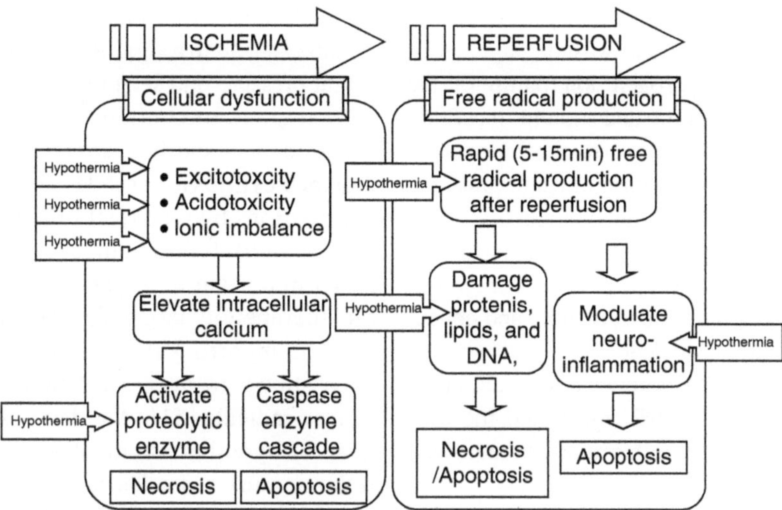

Fig. 3.1 Schematic illustrating the mechanisms of ischemic/reperfusional I/R injury and the effects of therapeutic hypothermia. We illustrate the potential mechanisms of ischemic/reperfusional (I/R) brain injury and the effective point of hypothermia treatment. The pathology of I/R injury is approximately separated as two mechanisms, i.e., the cell death following cellular dysfunction in ischemic phase, and the free radical production in reperfusion phase. The boxed arrow with entered "Hypothermia" means the estimated effective points in the I/R cascade

pump. This causes depolarization of the cell membrane leading to activation of voltage-gated calcium channels and an influx of intracellular calcium [34]. Moreover, with the anaerobic metabolism induced, intracellular and extracellular acidosis contributes to the calcium influx. This rapid increase in intracellular calcium causes the release of large amounts of the excitatory neurotransmitter glutamate, which further stimulates calcium influx in post-synaptic cells [35]. Among other things, calcium triggers activation of phospholipase, nitric oxide synthase, proteases, endonucleases, and oxidase enzymes [36]. These activated molecules can easily damage other cell proteins and lipid membranes causing necrosis [37]. Recent studies have also demonstrated the production of superoxide radicals by N-methyl-D-aspartate (NMDA) receptor-mediated nicotinamide adenine dinucleotide phosphate (NADPH) oxidase activation [38]. Such events amplify reactive oxygen species (ROS) production, mitochondrial dysfunction, and proapoptotic protein activation. Intracellular calcium accumulation itself also triggers initiation of mitochondrial dysfunction and fragmentation leading to activation of proapoptotic proteins such as the caspases [39].

Reperfusion to this ischemic tissue results in a short period of excessive free radical production [40]. Experimental measurements of the reperfusion phase demonstrate that oxygen- and carbon-centered free radicals peak within 5 min of reperfusion [41] and that hydroxyl generation peaks within 15 min [42]. This oxidative stress can damage proteins, lipids, and DNA, possibly leading to necrosis and apoptosis [43, 44]. Oxidants also modulate neuro-inflammation [45] leading to increased levels of neuronal apoptosis in adjacent cells [46–48].

Similar to findings with cerebral ischemia, several mechanisms of myocardial damage due to ischemia and reperfusion have been identified and investigated [24]. One potential mediator of lethal reperfusion injury in the heart also includes oxidative stress. Under normal circumstances, nitric oxide (NO) helps regulate the inhibition of neutrophil accumulation, inactivation of superoxide radicals, and coronary blood flow. However, during reperfusion injury, subsequent oxide stress leads to a diminished NO content and an increased accumulation of neutrophils and superoxide radicals. With oxidative stress, intracellular calcium overload also occurs due to sarcolemmal damage with resultant cardiomyocyte death. Rapid restoration of physiologic pH following lactic acid washout and activation of the sodium-hydrogen ion pump of the sodium-hydrogen ion pump and sodium- bicarbonate channel protein contribute to the reperfusion injury, as does the accumulation of neutrophils and inflammatory mediators. It is thought that these effects result in the opening of mitochondrial permeability transition pores leading to subsequent hypercontracture, neutrophil attraction, and enhancement of cardiomyocyte death.

In Fig. 3.1, we illustrate several potential of mechanisms underlying I/R injury and the estimated points where hypothermia treatment can effect.

Therapeutic Intervention: Hypothermia Therapy

Despite much basic and clinical research using hypothermia in I/R injury, the mechanisms of its neuronal protection remain unclear. To date, several mechanisms have been proposed to explain how therapeutic hypothermia provides protection against injury in various organ systems. Within the neural tissues, the cerebral metabolic rate determines perfusion. At colder temperatures, cerebral tissues require less perfusion, and this rate decreases by 6–7% for every 1°C decrease in temperature [16]. The immediate deficit in oxygen, adenosine triphosphate, and glucose which exist during the period of cerebral ischemia is, in part, overcome by the decreased metabolism demand via therapeutic hypothermia.

As mentioned above, brain injury does not only occur as a result of hypo-perfusion, but also with reperfusion. Nonetheless, the resultant reduction in oxygen consumption, the decrease in destructive cytotoxic cascades such as neutrophil transmigration, a reduction in excitatory amino acids that activate free radicals and nitric oxide (NO), a reduction in acidosis and maintenance of the blood–brain barrier, all support the reduction of tissue damage at the molecular level due to therapeutic hypothermia effect [11].

In the latter phase of cerebral ischemia, therapeutic hypothermia slows the deterioration of the blood–brain barrier, decreasing cerebral edema, which can lead to a significant reduction in intracranial pressure and seizure risk [33, 49, 50].

Mediators of continued ischemia which are released post cardiac arrest and activate and enhance cytotoxic cascades, are also limited in their actions by the effect of hypothermia [33]. Mitochondrial free radical production might be an important target and it provides a possible therapeutic target for hypothermia treatment. Supporting this point hypothermia has been shown to decrease abnormal production of free radicals [51]. Another potential mechanism of hypothermia involves the reduction of inflammatory cascades and cell death pathways of apoptosis and necrosis [52].

Hypothermia also reduces cellular metabolism and oxygen demand while maintaining acceptable ATP levels [53]. Likewise, it improves cellular ion handling and cellular pH balance [33].

One mechanism by which reperfusion causes myocardial damage is a phenomenon known as post ischemic reactive hyperemia, whereby following reperfusion, a dramatic rise in coronary circulation occurs, well above the normal flow prior to occlusion. A similar phenomenon has been described after a period of cerebral ischemia.

Therapeutic Interventions: Drugs and Chemical Agents

Previous work by Ames et al. describing a “no-reflow phenomena” in the reperfusioned brain provided a vascular target to possibly improve outcome [21]. This syndrome, quantitatively verified by other researchers [54–56], consists of reactive hyperemia during the first 5 min of reperfusion followed by a progressive and prolonged decline in cerebral blood flow. After 12–20 min of brain ischemia and 40–60 min reperfusion, flow is 20% of normal, a level below that required for neuronal survival. This occurs despite adequate perfusion pressures and is not related to intravascular clotting or increased intracranial pressure [55–57]. The mechanism of this phenomenon is thought to be calcium dependent. In the brain, equilibrium between the intra and extracellular components occurs during the first 5 min of the insult. As a result, rapid shifts of calcium into arterial walls occur and are accompanied by vascular spasm [58]. Based on these observations, calcium antagonists have been classically used to prevent further reperfusion injury. A similar no-reflow phenomenon occurs in the MI [59] and possibly in other tissues and organs as well. There was some evidence that the calcium antagonist diltiazem protects the myocardium during reperfusion [60]. However, with other experimental and clinical study, it was revealed that only part of the excessive uptake of calcium during the reperfusion period was susceptible to inhibition by calcium antagonists [61], and the increase of calcium during reperfusion could not be adequately prevented by calcium antagonists, at least not in pharmacologic dose [62]. Currently, several pathways of calcium transport have been investigated [63], and many candidates of drug therapy for reperfusion injury are still being studied in experimental and clinical investigations, i.e., not only L-type Ca^{2+} channel (LTCC) blocker [64–69], but also Na^+/Ca^{2+} exchanger (NCX) inhibitor [70–73] and Na^+/H^+ exchanger (NHE) inhibitor [74–78].

In animal experimental models, there is another important proposed mechanism: the formation of free radicals [79]. In experimental models, there is a evidence that free radical scavengers can decrease some degrees of reperfusion damage [80–85], however these effect are still un-known in clinical situations [86–88]. Especially in cardiac arrest experimental model, some agents of free radical scavenger have been also researched [89–91]. In conclusion, we have no definitive pharmacological treatment for reperfusion injury.

Therapeutic Interventions: Combination of Temperature Managements and Pharmacological Approaches

Mild therapeutic hypothermia following cardiac arrest is neuroprotective. However, to appreciate the maximum benefits of hypothermia therapy, hypothermia needs to be initiated as soon as possible after the insult and maintained for relatively long periods. Therapeutic hypothermia alone still has its limitations, and it might be advantageous to combine cooling with other treatment strategies. To increase protection and use of hypothermia, combination therapies including hypothermia and a second neuroprotectant have been investigated.

The addition of a secondary neuroprotectant has been aimed for enhancement of overall protection, prolonging of the therapeutic time window, and protection where hypothermia treatment is only transient [92]. Also, some pharmacological agents have been studied as a kind of preconditioning cardioprotectants with mild hypothermia therapy [93, 94].

The synergistic effects of combination therapy in ischemic experiments was first described by the combination of magnesium, tirilazad and hypothermia therapy [95–97]. Another combination method is that of caffeine and ethanol, or caffeinol [98] and therapeutic hypothermia. A clinical study of combination therapy with hypothermia, rt-PA and caffeinol is ongoing, and is perhaps the first clinical combination study of hypothermia and a pharmacological neuroprotectant in stroke patients. Preliminary reports in 20 patients indicate that this approach is feasible [99]. A prospective randomized study will be needed to further assess feasibility and to describe the efficacy of caffeinol, hypothermia, or both.

To extend the therapeutic window of mild hypothermia, other agents have been studied for combination therapy. FK 506 (Tacrolims) is one of these agents which may prolong therapeutic time windows. The therapeutic window for FK 506 treatment in cerebral ischemia was estimated to be greater than 1 h, but less than 2 h. Combining this pharmacological treatment with hypothermia led to an elongation of the temporary therapeutic window to 2 h [100].

Combinational treatment of a neuroprotectant with hypothermia can also sustain protection, where hypothermic protection was previously found to be only transient. Some experiments have shown that post ischemic hypothermic protection with cooling for 3 h is transient following forebrain ischemia [101]. However, if hypothermia is followed by the injection of the MK-801(NMDA antagonist) on specific post ischemic periods, animals showed longer neurological protection out to 6–8 weeks [102].

Further, mild hypothermia (induced as 33–34°C immediately on reperfusion for 4 h) has also been combined with anti-inflammatory cytokine IL-10 given in the immediate post ischemic period. In this study, histological protection in hippocampus CAI could be shown to last up to 2 months [103].

In experimental cardiac arrest models, combination therapies have also been studied. Mild hypothermia was induced in the early reperfusion phase with a post conditioning therapy (inhalation of Xenon or sevoflurane, a volatile anesthetic agent). The combination of 20% xenon and hypothermia of 34°C, applied during early reperfusion, reduced infarct size in the rat heart in vivo [94]. Also, hypothermia and post conditioning with sevoflurane reduced cardiac dysfunction by modulating inflammation, apoptosis and remodeling [93, 104]. However, experimental settings employing hypothermia in combination with sevoflurane showed that the volatile anesthetic agent did not confer additional anti-inflammatory effects in the cerebral cortex of pigs after cardiopulmonary resuscitation [104].

From the previous data regarding combination therapy in clinical and experimental studies, it was suggested that the combination therapy might be safe and warranted in some clinical conditions. However, more clinical and experimental studies should be needed in this topic.

Therapeutic Hypothermia in Myocardial Infarction

Many studies have demonstrated the efficacy of therapeutic hypothermia on neurologic outcomes [12, 105, 106]. However, until recently, there has not been much evidence regarding the effects of therapeutic hypothermia on the heart itself, particularly its potential to decrease MI size.

Many experiments relating the effectiveness of therapeutic hypothermia in MI have been conducted. In a rat experimental model, Miki et al. studied the effect of hypothermia on cardiomyocytes with a MI model [8]. They clarified that therapeutic hypothermia to 32°C significantly delayed the appearance of both cellular osmotic fragility and cellular contracture, and concluded that mild hypothermia could delay the onset of I/R injury in cardiomyocytes.

Mild hypothermia also has been shown in animal studies to limit the size of AMI, Abendschien et al. examined whether hypothermia (26°C) affected infarct size in experimental model subjected to a 5-h left anterior descending coronary artery occlusion without subsequent reperfusion after 30 min of occlusion. The investigators measured postmortem MI area and observed that infarct size in dogs receiving hypothermia was significantly reduced compared to normothermia treatment [107]. Abendschien et al. concluded that therapeutic hypothermia might be a useful in clinical myocardial revascularization.

Several translational clinical trials have investigated the feasibility and efficacy of therapeutic hypothermia for the treatment of persisting I/R injury in MI. Feasibility and safety trials include Noninvasive cooling for Acute Myocardial Infarction (NICAMI, surface cooling) [108, 109], and lowering Adverse Outcomes with Temperature Regulation Feasibility (LOWTEMP, endovascular cooling) [109].

Randomized controlled trials have also been conducted including the COOL MI and the ICE-IT trials. Unfortunately, these two trials showed negative results [110–112]. In both trials, there were problems with achieving target temperature before reperfusion. On the other hand, patients who reached target temperature demonstrated significant reductions in infarct size, especially for anterior infarcts [24].

Mild hypothermia for MI is a very potent cardio protective treatment, at least in the experimental setting. The benefit depends upon the timing with which cooling is instituted and by how much it shortens the normothermiac ischemic time. To afford a clinical benefit, a cooling strategy should accordingly be intended to reach the target temperature well before the time of revascularization. More clinical studies of early induced mild hypothermia are needed to determine their effectiveness for myocardial protection against I/R injury.

Therapeutic Hypothermia for Cardiac Arrest

In animal models of cardiac arrest, stores of oxygen in the brain are lost in seconds, and stores of glucose and ATP are lost within 5 min [113, 114]. Hypoxia and substrate depletion quickly lead to the loss of transmembrane electrochemical gradients and subsequent failure of synaptic transmission, axonal conduction, and action-potential firing [115]. Glutamate, which is the major excitatory neurotransmitter, is released and intracellular calcium accumulates, leading to excitotoxic cell death [116, 117]. Several regions of the brain are especially vulnerable to a global ischemic insult including the CA1 hippocampus, neocortex, cerebellum, corpus striatum, and thalamus [118]. Both necrosis and apoptosis in neural tissues have been reported after cardiac arrest, although the degree of contribution in the cell death to the resulting brain injury remains unclear [119].

After restoration of blood flow, reperfusion and reoxygenation can lead to further neuronal damage in several hours to days, and this continues to the reperfusion injury [105]. Cerebral microcirculatory failure associated with initial periods of transient global hyperemia due to dysfunction of vascular autoregulation along with prolonged hypoperfusion have been described [120]. Re-oxygenation initiates complex chemical cascades producing free radicals that cause lipid peroxydation and other oxidative damage [121]. Alterations in the inflammatory response also can cause endothelial cell activation, leukocyte infiltration, and further tissue injury [45]. Other contributing factors, including hypotension, hypoxemia, impaired cerebrovascular autoregulation, and brain edema, can all further interrupt the delivery of oxygen to the brain and return of normal function.

Hypothermia therapy has therefore been targeted to these mechanisms of injury, and much basic research has been performed. In human studies, hypothermia caused a reduction in brain metabolism, including a reduction in oxygen utilization and ATP consumption [122]. Hypothermia also inhibited the extracellular release glutamate and dopamine and induced brain derived neurotrophic factor expression, which further reduced the release of glutamate [123, 124]. Oxidative stress is attenuated with hypothermic treatment and lipid peroxydation is also reduced [125, 126]. Apoptosis is initiated as a result of a reduction in calcium overload and glutamate release. Hypothermia can reduce apoptotic cell death by the induction of antiapoptotic Bcl-2 and the suppression of the proapoptotic factor BAX [127]. Hypothermia has also been shown to reduce the inflammation that occurs after ischemia [128] and to reduce both early hyperemia and delayed hypoperfusion [129].

The temperature management trials that provided strong evidence in clinical situations with mild hypothermia management were published in 2002 [11, 12]. These two trials have become the basis of clinical guidelines regarding the use of therapeutic hypothermia for cardiac arrest patients. In the trial conducted in Australia, 77 comatose survivors of cardiac arrest, whose initial cardiac rhythms were ventricular fibrillation (VF), were enrolled [12] to cooling protocol of 33°C, 12 h duration. Hypothermia-induced patients had more favorable outcomes (49%) at the time of discharge than that of normothemia-induced patients (26%, P=0.05). The odds ratio for a favorable neurologic recovery with hypothermia therapy was 5.25 (95% CI; 1.47–18.76, P-0.01), after adjustment for age and duration of the arrest.

In another multicenter trial held in Europe, 275 comatose survivors of a cardiac arrest of cardiac cause (VF or pulseless ventricular tachycardia) were enrolled [11]. Patients were randomly assigned to the hypothermia group (32–34°C, 24 h duration) or to normothermia as standard treatment. 55% of the hypothermia group had a better neurologic recovery after 6 months, as compared with 39% in the normothermia group. In addition, as compared with standard treatment with normothermia, there was a significant reduction with hypothemia in mortality at 6 months (risk ratio for death, 0.74; 95% CI, 0.58–0.95). With these strong findings from two clinical studies, mild hypothermia for cardiac arrest patients has gained worldwide use as a method of treating this patient population [99, 130–132].

Therapeutic Hypothermia for Cerebral Infarction

Many animal studies have indicated the efficacy of hypothermia in ischemic stroke. Van der Worp et al. performed a meta-analysis on the efficacy of hypothermia in rat models of ischemic stroke [133]. In this review, the effectiveness was noted by the reduction of infarct size and improvement of outcome. These results indicated a 44% reduction in infarct size (95%CI 40–47%) at a target temperature of 35°C when the initiation of treatment occurred between 90 and 180 min after artery occlusion. Potentially, these results may have significant consequences for the treatment of large numbers of patients with acute ischemic stroke.

However, the successful translation of preclinical data to human studies has not been easy due to small numbers of participants and varying methods and measurements, making comparisons difficult. In eight recent cooling therapy trials for acute ischemic stroke involving a total of 423 patients [134], a meta-analysis of pharmacological and physical temperature reduction trials indicated no significant difference between the active treatment group and the control group with regard to primary outcomes of death or dependency at 1 or 3 months after stroke (OR=0.9, 95% CI=0.6–1.4).

The Intravascular Cooling in the Treatment of Strole-Longer Window (ICTuS-L) trial was recently completed [6]. This trial investigated the combination of intravenous tissue plasminogen activator/alteplase (tPA) and intravascular hypothermia after ischemic stroke. In this trial, hypothermia treatment did not have a significant effect on Mortality or morbidity at 3 months. Symptomatic hemorrhage occurred in four patients, all of whom received tPA less than 3 h, one of whom additionally received hypothermia treatment. Pneumonia was reported in 14 patients who received hypothermia treatment versus 3 in the normothermia group, however, this did not adversely affect disability outcomes. Importantly, this study showed some degree of safety and feasibility with the use of hypothermia as a neuroprotective therapy in stroke.

Neuroprotective strategies after ischemic stroke remain a promising field for investigating novel therapeutic interventions. Hypothermia is the strongest neuroprotective therapy in experimental ischemia studies. Advances in hypothermia delivery using endovascular heat exchanges and novel anti-shivering protocols are improving the routine clinical use of hypothermia after ischemic stroke [135]. Studies are ongoing to investigate the effect of hypothermia in other clinical situations. Further innovations will continue to include combining hypothermia with thrombolysis and other neuroprotective strategies.

Therapeutic Hypothermia for Traumatic Brain Injury

Ischemic mechanisms have been considered to participate in the pathophysiology of traumatic brain injury (TBI). In this regard, both primary and secondary brain injury mechanisms may be related to ischemic insults. For example, in a severe fluid percussion injury rat model, Dietrich et al. revealed the severe reduction of local cerebral blood flow in the posttraumatic phase with an autoradiographic and histopathological study [136]. Also in the posttraumatic phase, systemic hypotension has been reported to deteriorate the cerebral ischemic insult and worsen outcome following brain injury [137]. To mitigate this secondary ischemic insult, posttraumatic hypothermia therapy has been said to be effective in several models [138].

I/R pathophysiology in TBI patients was first described by Muizellar et al. The group used stable Xenon-computed tomography and measured cerebral blood flow in 26 traumatic head injury patients [139]. From these results they concluded that I/R pathophysiology was a significant part of certain traumatic brain injuries.

In 1990, ischemic brain damage was first described in the ASDH rat model by Miller, et al. They injected autologous blood into the subdural space and induced ASDH. They confirmed the ischemic change with histological assessment [140]. Kuroda and Bullock also used a similar ASDH model to autoradiographically map regional cerebral blood flow before and after removal of hematoma. They concluded that a major cause of hemisphere swelling, seen after hematoma removal, was due to enlargement of the zone experiencing focal tissue ischemia occurring just beneath the hematoma, and that neuronal damage continued even after decompressive craniotomy [141]. Epidural hematomas are related to this I/R pathophysiology as well. In one experimental study, a rat epidural balloon compression model was used and researchers examined a variety of outcome measures including cerebral blood flow (CBF) measured with laser Doppler flowmetry, brain tissue oxygenation ($PtiO_2$), magnetic resonance imaging, and histological changes in brain tissue. In the time period during balloon inflation, the value of CBF and $PtiO_2$ decreased, recovering with balloon deflation. This study also demonstrated that intra-ischemic hypothermia might reduce the ischemia-induced tissue damage and hippocampal neuronal cell injury [142].

The evidence from these previous reports allows us to conclude that traumatic focal brain injury concurrent with evacuated mass lesions, i.e., subdural or epidural hematomas, represents an I/R injury.

Previous clinical trials in TBI have been unable to establish the efficacy of hypothermia although several institutional trials have reported benefits. In a multicenter trial using hypothermia as an intervention [143], 392 patients with acute brain injury were randomized to normothermia or surface-induced hypothermia groups. Unfortunately, no improvement in outcome was noted between temperature groups (the National Acute Brain Injury Study: Hypothermia, NABIS: H). However, there was some weak evidence of improved outcomes in patients who were hypothermic on admission and treated with continued hypothermia [143]. This same study group then tried to determine the efficacy of very early hypothermia in patients with severe brain injury; the National Acute Brain Injury Study: Hypothermia II (NABIS: H II) [144]. In NABIS: H II, the early-induced hypothermia similarly did not demonstrate efficacy when researchers looked at mortality and morbidity data. On the other hand, in a sub-population analysis that divided the diffuse brain injury patients and those with surgical hematoma evacuation, early-induced hypothermia proved efficacious for the later group (poor outcome ratio; 33% in hypothermia group vs. 69% in normothermia group, $P=0.02$). The authors concluded that one explanation was the different pathophysiology between diffuse brain injury and hematoma. As mentioned above, ischemia occurs during ASDH expansion followed by reperfusion injury after removal [139, 141]. This injury has similar pathophysiological mechanisms of injury to that seen in patients with cardiac arrest—a group that has been successfully treated with hypothermia [10]. As mentioned previously, encouraging experimental data demonstrated that intra-ischemic hypothermia prior to hematoma removal was associated with improved outcome [142]. Diffuse brain injury is not characterized by ischemia in in-vitro studies and would therefore not be a good candidate for hypothermia treatment [145]. The authors of NABIS: H II concluded that their finding of improved outcome in patients with evacuated hematomas warranted further study.

Therapeutic Hypothermia for Decompression Surgery

The efficacy of combination therapy of therapeutic hypothermia and decompression surgery is not well studied. In one investigation using a focal ischemia rat model, a combination of decompressive craniotomy and mild hypothermia (32°C) induction upregulated the expression of Bcl-2 (antiapoptotic protein) and downregulates the expression of Bax (proapoptotic protein). This result may indicate that the combination therapy of therapeutic mild hypothermia and decompressive craniotomy might reduce cell apoptosis. Interestingly, this experiment also reported the reduction of the infarct size after permanent focal cerebral ischemia in rats [146].

As mentioned above, The ASDH patients with removed hematomas has I/R pathophysiology [141], and the latest clinical study revealed that early-induced, pre-reperfusional induced hypothermia might be effective in this subgroup of patients. Hypothesizing that hypothermia would reduce neuronal death in ASDH by blunting the effects of reperfusion injury, we initiated a pilot study and conducted basic experimental research using a well established rat model [140, 141]. In our experiment, 40 rats were induced with ASDH and placed into one of four groups; (1) the normothermia group was maintained at 37°C throughout the experiment, (2) the early hypothermia group was cooled to 33°C at 30 min prior to craniotomy and kept at this temperature for 3 h afterward, (3) the late hypothermia group was cooled to 33°C at 30 min after decompressive craniotomy and kept at this temperature for 3 h, and (4) the sham group who received no ASDH induction and underwent only craniotomy with normothermia. For estimation of neuronal cell damage, we analyzed microdialysate (MD; using 100kD probe) concentrations of ubiquitin carboxyl-terminal hydrolase -L1 (UCH-L1) as a biomarker of neuronal injury [147, 148]. We also quantified the volume of infarction by 2,3,5-triphenyltetrazolium chloride (TTC) staining, using a previously described technique [149, 150]. We then analyzed these variables and compared them between the different treatment groups. Results from preliminary data show that early-induced hypothermia reduces the concentration of MD UCH-L1 (Fig. 3.2) and the volume of ischemia as measured by TTC (Fig. 3.3a–c). These novel data indicate that early induced hypothermia may reduce neural cell damage and injured volume in ASDH rat model.

Based on the results from this animal study and the clinical results from the NABIS: H II, a large multicenter clinical trial is warranted to further investigate the effect of early hypothermia in I/R traumatic brain injury.

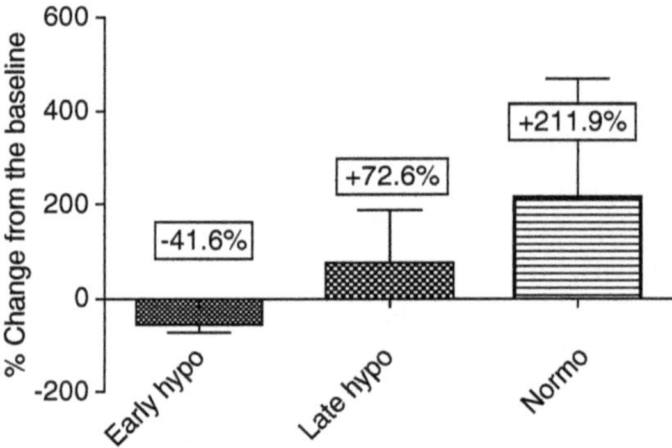

Fig. 3.2 Relative change (%) of UCH-L1 Md concentration from baseline after a decompressive craniotomy. This graph shows the relative ratio of ubiquitin carboxyl-terminal hydrolase -L1 concentration in microdialysates (UCH-L1 MD) from baseline (pre-craniotomy) levels. A significantly negative ratio was observed in only the early-induced hypothermia group. In the late induced hypothermia and normothermia groups, the relative ratios were positive. *Early Hypo* early hypothermia therapy, *Late Hypo* late hypothermia therapy, *Normo* normothermia therapy

Future Directions

Although therapeutic hypothermia has been shown in multicenter trials to benefit patients with cardiac arrest and term babies with hypoxic insults, much work is required to determine what other patient populations may benefit from this exciting treatment. Since the pathophysiology of I/R brain injury might be similar in other pathological conditions, mild hypothermia therapy might be a valuable option for a broader population of patients. There are several factors that play an important role in whether hypothermia is protective. The appropriate timing and methods to induce hypothermia, the effective level and duration of hypothermia and the optimal length of time to target temperature reductions all may significantly contribute to long term outcomes. In this regard, the potential effect of the rate of rewarming on neurologic outcome after cardiac arrest is still unknown. In future investigations, more information regarding these components of temperature management may provide the necessary information that would allow for better

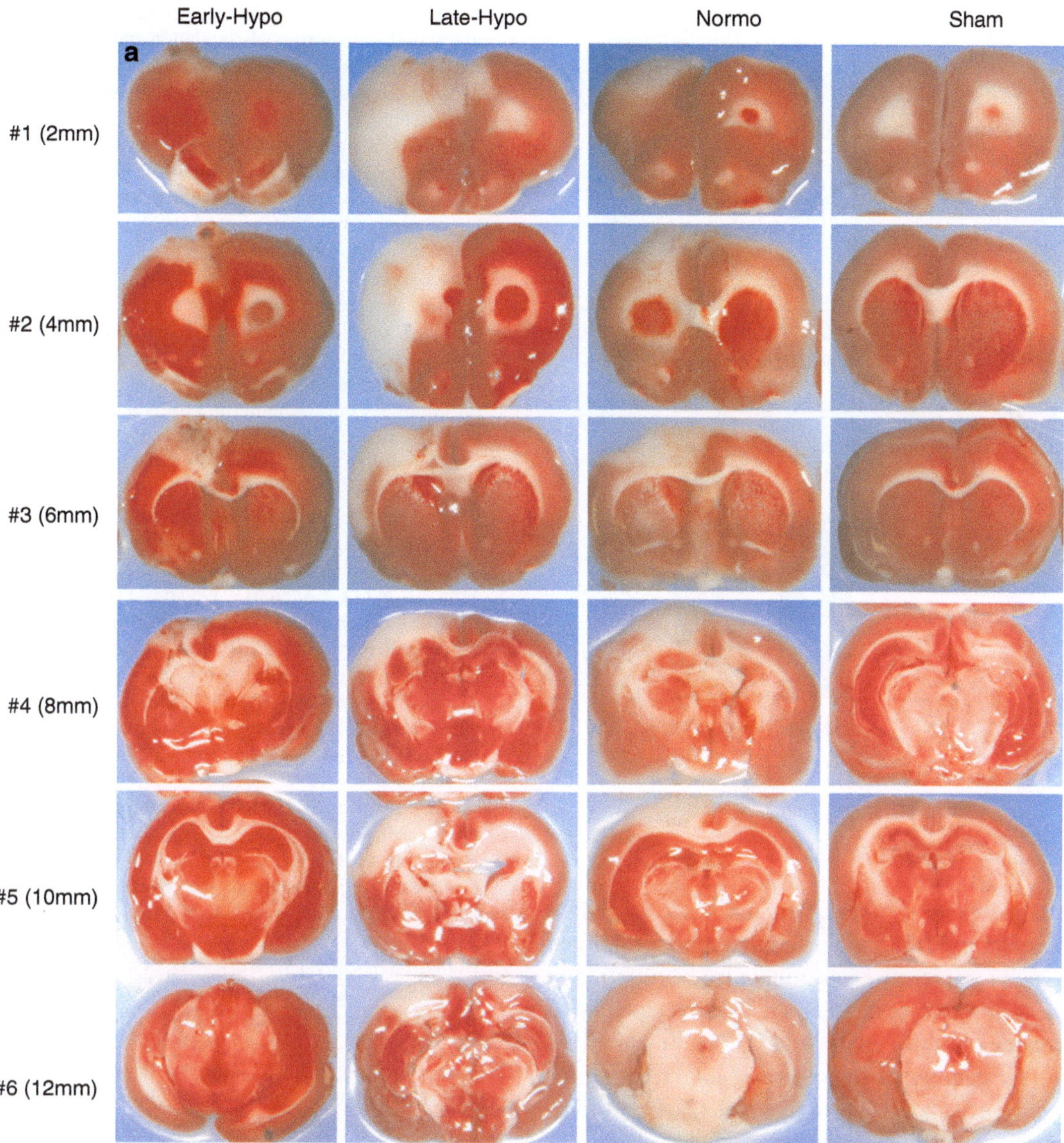

Fig. 3.3 TTC (2,3,5-triphenyltetrazolium chloride) ischemic volumetry in each treatment group. (**a**) TTC staining of ischemic areas: after decompressive craniotomy following ASDA induction 2 mm thick sections were made throughout the forebrain of the injured animals. Using this methodology, regions of ischemic/damage were identified as unstained, white areas. In sham rats, no evidence of ischemic regions was observed. Also, in animals where hypothermia was initiated prior to decompression surgery, small well defined unstained areas were commonly seen. In contrast, the late induced hypothermia and normothermia groups both demonstrated larger ischemic lesions throughout the forebrain structures. *Early-Hypo* early induced hypothermia group, *Late-Hypo* late induced hypothermia group, *Normo* normothermia group. (**b**) Ischemic area measurements. This graph shows the percentage of ischemic area (percentage which defined as ratio of injury area/total area). In the early induced hypothermia group, the area of ischemic injury was reduced compared to that seen in the normothermic or in the delayed hypothermic groups (N=5 each, $^*P<0.05$, with unpaired *T* test). (**c**) Ischemic volumes: we compared the absolute ischemic volumes among the three treatment groups (N=5 each). In the early, preoperative- induced hypothermia group, ischemic area was significantly reduced compare to the other two groups (one-way ANOVA P=0.0137, $^*P<0.05$, with Tukey-Kramer post-hoc test). *E-Hypo* early hypothermia therapy, *L-Hypo* late hypothermia therapy, *Normo* normothermia therapy

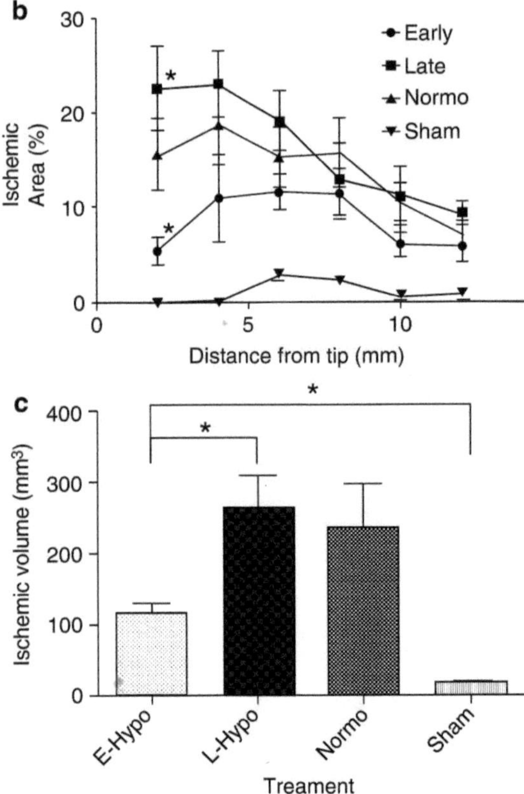

Fig. 3.3 (continued)

treatments to the tested in our various patient populations. It is anticipated that more prolonged hypothermia treatments might also be required in the setting of severe injury, as advocated with previous studies in rodents [151]. In addition, milder degrees of hypothermia might have protective effects similar to those of the target temperatures used in current protocols [152].

Further clinical study should also continue to evaluate combination therapies (mild hypothermia+pharmacological agent, mild hypothermia+decompression surgery, etc.). It will be important to determine what co-treatments should be combined to potentially produce synergic benefits to the patients.

References

1. Lewis FJ. Hypothermia in cardiac and general surgery. Minn Med. 1955;38:77–81.
2. Sealy WC, Brown Jr IW, Young Jr WG. A report on the use of both extracorporeal circulation and hypothermia for open heart surgery. Ann Surg. 1958;147:603–13.
3. Swan H. Hypothermia for general and cardiac surgery; with techniques of some open intracardiac procedures under hypothermia. Surg Clin North Am. 1956:1009–24.
4. Moossa AR, Zarins CK, Skinner DB. In situ kidney preservation for transplantation with use of profound hypothermia (5 to 20 degrees C.) with an intact circulation. Surgery. 1976;79:60–4.
5. De Georgia MA, Krieger DW, Abou-Chebl A, et al. Cooling for Acute Ischemic Brain Damage (COOL AID): a feasibility trial of endovascular cooling. Neurology. 2004;63:312–7.
6. Hemmen TM, Raman R, Guluma KZ, et al. Intravenous thrombolysis plus hypothermia for acute treatment of ischemic stroke (ICTuS-L): final results. Stroke. 2010; 41:2265–70.
7. Dae MW, Gao DW, Sessler DI, Chair K, Stillson CA. Effect of endovascular cooling on myocardial temperature, infarct size, and cardiac output in human-sized pigs. Am J Physiol Heart Circ Physiol. 2002;282:H1584–91.
8. Miki T, Liu GS, Cohen MV, Downey JM. Mild hypothermia reduces infarct size in the beating rabbit heart: a practical intervention for acute myocardial infarction? Basic Res Cardiol. 1998;93:372–83.
9. Abella BS, Zhao D, Alvarado J, Hamann K, Vanden Hoek TL, Becker LB. Intra-arrest cooling improves outcomes in a murine cardiac arrest model. Circulation. 2004;109:2786–91.
10. Janata A, Holzer M. Hypothermia after cardiac arrest. Prog Cardiovasc Dis. 2009;52:168–79.
11. Hypothermia after Cardiac Arrest Study Group. Mild therapeutic hypothermia to improve the neurologic outcome after cardiac arrest. N Engl J Med. 2002; 346:549–56.
12. Bernard SA, Gray TW, Buist MD, et al. Treatment of comatose survivors of out-of-hospital cardiac arrest with induced hypothermia. N Engl J Med. 2002;346: 557–63.
13. Tissier R, Hamanaka K, Kuno A, Parker JC, Cohen MV, Downey JM. Total liquid ventilation provides ultra-fast cardioprotective cooling. J Am Coll Cardiol. 2007;49:601–5.
14. Olivecrona GK, Gotberg M, Harnek J, Van der Pals J, Erlinge D. Mild hypothermia reduces cardiac post-ischemic reactive hyperemia. BMC Cardiovasc Disord. 2007;7:5.
15. Weisser J, Martin J, Bisping E, et al. Influence of mild hypothermia on myocardial contractility and circulatory function. Basic Res Cardiol. 2001;96:198–205.
16. Azmoon S, Demarest C, Pucillo AL, et al. Neurologic and cardiac benefits of therapeutic hypothermia. Cardiol Rev. 2011;19:108–14.
17. Heiss WD, Rosner G. Functional recovery of cortical neurons as related to degree and duration of ischemia. Ann Neurol. 1983;14:294–301.
18. Reimer KA, Jennings RB. The "wavefront phenomenon" of myocardial ischemic cell death. II. Transmural progression of necrosis within the framework of

ischemic bed size (myocardium at risk) and collateral flow. Lab Invest. 1979;40:633–44.
19. Braunwald E, Kloner RA. Myocardial reperfusion: a double-edged sword? J Clin Invest. 1985;76: 1713–9.
20. Hallenbeck JM, Dutka AJ. Background review and current concepts of reperfusion injury. Arch Neurol. 1990;47:1245–54.
21. Ames 3rd A, Wright RL, Kowada M, Thurston JM, Majno G. Cerebral ischemia. II. The no-reflow phenomenon. Am J Pathol. 1968;52:437–53.
22. Dietrich WD. Morphological manifestations of reperfusion injury in brain. Ann N Y Acad Sci. 1994; 723:15–24.
23. Jennings RB, Sommers HM, Smyth GA, Flack HA, Linn H. Myocardial necrosis induced by temporary occlusion of a coronary artery in the dog. Arch Pathol. 1960;70:68–78.
24. Yellon DM, Hausenloy DJ. Myocardial reperfusion injury. N Engl J Med. 2007;357:1121–35.
25. Braunwald E, Kloner RA. The stunned myocardium: prolonged, postischemic ventricular dysfunction. Circulation. 1982;66:1146–9.
26. Krug A, Du Mesnil de Rochemont R, Korb G. Blood supply of the myocardium after temporary coronary occlusion. Circ Res. 1966;19:57–62.
27. Ito H. No-reflow phenomenon and prognosis in patients with acute myocardial infarction. Nat Clin Pract Cardiovasc Med. 2006;3:499–506.
28. Manning AS, Hearse DJ. Reperfusion-induced arrhythmias: mechanisms and prevention. J Mol Cell Cardiol. 1984;16:497–518.
29. Kloner RA. Does reperfusion injury exist in humans? J Am Coll Cardiol. 1993;21:537–45.
30. Piper HM, Garcia-Dorado D, Ovize M. A fresh look at reperfusion injury. Cardiovasc Res. 1998;38:291–300.
31. Yellon DM, Baxter GF. Reperfusion injury revisited: is there a role for growth factor signaling in limiting lethal reperfusion injury? Trends Cardiovasc Med. 1999;9:245–9.
32. Lampe JW, Becker LB. State of the art in therapeutic hypothermia. Annu Rev Med. 2011;62:79–93.
33. Polderman KH. Mechanisms of action, physiological effects, and complications of hypothermia. Crit Care Med. 2009;37:S186–202.
34. Badruddin A, Taqi MA, Abraham MG, Dani D, Zaidat OO. Neurocritical care of a reperfused brain. Curr Neurol Neurosci Rep. 2011;11:104–10.
35. Simon RP. Acidotoxicity trumps excitotoxicity in ischemic brain. Arch Neurol. 2006;63:1368–71.
36. Wahlgren NG, Ahmed N. Neuroprotection in cerebral ischaemia: facts and fancies – the need for new approaches. Cerebrovasc Dis. 2004;17 Suppl 1: 153–66.
37. Leker RR, Shohami E. Cerebral ischemia and trauma-different etiologies yet similar mechanisms: neuroprotective opportunities. Brain Res Brain Res Rev. 2002;39:55–73.
38. Brennan AM, Suh SW, Won SJ, et al. NADPH oxidase is the primary source of superoxide induced by NMDA receptor activation. Nat Neurosci. 2009; 12:857–63.
39. Eldadah BA, Faden AI. Caspase pathways, neuronal apoptosis, and CNS injury. J Neurotrauma. 2000;17: 811–29.
40. Tuttolomondo A, Di Sciacca R, Di Raimondo D, et al. Neuron protection as a therapeutic target in acute ischemic stroke. Curr Top Med Chem. 2009;9: 1317–34.
41. Bolli R, Jeroudi MO, Patel BS, et al. Marked reduction of free radical generation and contractile dysfunction by antioxidant therapy begun at the time of reperfusion. Evidence that myocardial "stunning" is a manifestation of reperfusion injury. Circ Res. 1989; 65:607–22.
42. Khalid MA, Ashraf M. Direct detection of endogenous hydroxyl radical production in cultured adult cardiomyocytes during anoxia and reoxygenation. Is the hydroxyl radical really the most damaging radical species? Circ Res. 1993;72:725–36.
43. Halliwell B. Free radicals, antioxidants, and human disease: curiosity, cause, or consequence? Lancet. 1994;344:721–4.
44. Sugawara T, Chan PH. Reactive oxygen radicals and pathogenesis of neuronal death after cerebral ischemia. Antioxid Redox Signal. 2003;5:597–607.
45. Wong CH, Crack PJ. Modulation of neuro-inflammation and vascular response by oxidative stress following cerebral ischemia-reperfusion injury. Curr Med Chem. 2008;15:1–14.
46. Huang Y, Rabb H, Womer KL. Ischemia-reperfusion and immediate T cell responses. Cell Immunol. 2007; 248:4–11.
47. Jung JE, Kim GS, Chen H, et al. Reperfusion and neurovascular dysfunction in stroke: from basic mechanisms to potential strategies for neuroprotection. Mol Neurobiol. 2010;41:172–9.
48. Lu XC, Hartings JA, Si Y, Balbir A, Cao Y, Tortella FC. Electrocortical pathology in a rat model of penetrating ballistic-like brain injury. J Neurotrauma. 2011; 28:71–83.
49. Bernard SA, Buist M. Induced hypothermia in critical care medicine: a review. Crit Care Med. 2003;31: 2041–51.
50. Howes D, Green R, Gray S, Stenstrom R, Easton D. Evidence for the use of hypothermia after cardiac arrest. CJEM. 2006;8:109–15.
51. Shao ZH, Sharp WW, Wojcik KR, et al. Therapeutic hypothermia cardioprotection via Akt- and nitric oxide-mediated attenuation of mitochondrial oxidants. Am J Physiol Heart Circ Physiol. 2010;298: H2164–73.
52. Yang D, Guo S, Zhang T, Li H. Hypothermia attenuates ischemia/reperfusion-induced endothelial cell apoptosis via alterations in apoptotic pathways and JNK signaling. FEBS Lett. 2009;583:2500–6.
53. Erecinska M, Thoresen M, Silver IA. Effects of hypothermia on energy metabolism in Mammalian central nervous system. J Cereb Blood Flow Metab. 2003;23: 513–30.

54. Gadzinski DS, White BC, Hoehner PJ, Hoehner T, Krome C, White JD. Canine cerebral cortical blood flow and vascular resistance post cardiac arrest. Ann Emerg Med. 1982;11:58–63.
55. Snyder JV, Nemoto EM, Carroll RG, Safar P. Global ischemia in dogs: intracranial pressures, brain blood flow and metabolism. Stroke. 1975;6:21–7.
56. Drewes LR, Gilboe DD, Betz AL. Metabolic alterations in brain during anoxic-anoxia and subsequent recovery. Arch Neurol. 1973;29:385–90.
57. Kowada M, Ames 3rd A, Majno G, Wright RL. Cerebral ischemia. I. An improved experimental method for study; cardiovascular effects and demonstration of an early vascular lesion in the rabbit. J Neurosurg. 1968;28:150–7.
58. Van Nueten JM, Vanhoutte PM. Improvement of tissue perfusion with inhibitors of calcium ion influx. Biochem Pharmacol. 1980;29:479–81.
59. Shen AC, Jennings RB. Myocardial calcium and magnesium in acute ischemic injury. Am J Pathol. 1972;67: 417–40.
60. Cavero I, Boudot JP, Feuvray D. Diltiazem protects the isolated rabbit heart from the mechanical and ultrastructural damage produced by transient hypoxia, low-flow ischemia and exposure to Ca++-free medium. J Pharmacol Exp Ther. 1983;226: 258–68.
61. Nayler WG, Ferrari R, Williams A. Protective effect of pretreatment with verapamil, nifedipine and propranolol on mitochondrial function in the ischemic and reperfused myocardium. Am J Cardiol. 1980;46: 242–8.
62. Nayler WG, Panagiotopoulos S, Elz JS, Daly MJ. Calcium-mediated damage during post-ischaemic reperfusion. J Mol Cell Cardiol. 1988;20 Suppl 2:41–54.
63. Talukder MA, Zweier JL, Periasamy M. Targeting calcium transport in ischaemic heart disease. Cardiovasc Res. 2009;84:345–52.
64. Dirksen MT, Laarman GJ, Simoons ML, Duncker DJ. Reperfusion injury in humans: a review of clinical trials on reperfusion injury inhibitory strategies. Cardiovasc Res. 2007;74:343–55.
65. Bush LR, Romson JL, Ash JL, Lucchesi BR. Effect of diltiazem on extent of ultimate myocardial injury resulting from temporary coronary artery occlusion in dogs. J Cardiovasc Pharmacol. 1982;4:285–96.
66. Standefer M, Little JR. Improved neurological outcome in experimental focal cerebral ischemia treated with propranolol. Neurosurgery. 1986;18:136–40.
67. Lamping KA, Gross GJ. Improved recovery of myocardial segment function following a short coronary occlusion in dogs by nicorandil, a potential new antianginal agent, and nifedipine. J Cardiovasc Pharmacol. 1985;7:158–66.
68. Przyklenk K, Ghafari GB, Eitzman DT, Kloner RA. Nifedipine administered after reperfusion ablates systolic contractile dysfunction of postischemic "stunned" myocardium. J Am Coll Cardiol. 1989;13: 1176–83.
69. Gross GJ, Farber NE, Pieper GM. Effects of amlodipine on myocardial ischemia-reperfusion injury in dogs. Am J Cardiol. 1989;64:94I–100.
70. Blaustein MP, Lederer WJ. Sodium/calcium exchange: its physiological implications. Physiol Rev. 1999;79: 763–854.
71. Ohtsuka M, Takano H, Suzuki M, et al. Role of Na^{+}-Ca^{2+} exchanger in myocardial ischemia/reperfusion injury: evaluation using a heterozygous Na^{+}-Ca^{2+} exchanger knockout mouse model. Biochem Biophys Res Commun. 2004;314:849–53.
72. Inserte J, Garcia-Dorado D, Ruiz-Meana M, et al. Effect of inhibition of Na(+)/Ca(2+) exchanger at the time of myocardial reperfusion on hypercontracture and cell death. Cardiovasc Res. 2002;55:739–48.
73. Vittone L, Mundina-Weilenmann C, Mattiazzi A. Phospholamban phosphorylation by CaMKII under pathophysiological conditions. Front Biosci. 2008;13:5988–6005.
74. Karmazyn M. Pharmacology and clinical assessment of cariporide for the treatment coronary artery diseases. Expert Opin Investig Drugs. 2000;9: 1099–108.
75. Avkiran M, Marber MS. Na(+)/H(+) exchange inhibitors for cardioprotective therapy: progress, problems and prospects. J Am Coll Cardiol. 2002;39:747–53.
76. Murphy E, Allen DG. Why did the NHE inhibitor clinical trials fail? J Mol Cell Cardiol. 2009;46: 137–41.
77. Shi Y, Chanana V, Watters JJ, Ferrazzano P, Sun D. Role of sodium/hydrogen exchanger isoform 1 in microglial activation and proinflammatory responses in ischemic brains. J Neurochem. 2011;119: 124–35.
78. Barry WH, Zhang XQ, Halkos ME, et al. Nonanticoagulant heparin reduces myocyte Na^{+} and Ca^{2+} loading during simulated ischemia and decreases reperfusion injury. Am J Physiol Heart Circ Physiol. 2010;298:H102–11.
79. Opie LH. Reperfusion injury and its pharmacologic modification. Circulation. 1989;80:1049–62.
80. Myers CL, Weiss SJ, Kirsh MM, Shlafer M. Involvement of hydrogen peroxide and hydroxyl radical in the 'oxygen paradox': reduction of creatine kinase release by catalase, allopurinol or deferoxamine, but not by superoxide dismutase. J Mol Cell Cardiol. 1985;17:675–84.
81. Ambrosio G, Weisfeldt ML, Jacobus WE, Flaherty JT. Evidence for a reversible oxygen radical-mediated component of reperfusion injury: reduction by recombinant human superoxide dismutase administered at the time of reflow. Circulation. 1987;75:282–91.
82. Bolli R, Patel BS, Jeroudi MO, Lai EK, McCay PB. Demonstration of free radical generation in "stunned" myocardium of intact dogs with the use of the spin trap alpha-phenyl N-tert-butyl nitrone. J Clin Invest. 1988;82:476–85.
83. Bolli R, Zhu WX, Hartley CJ, et al. Attenuation of dysfunction in the postischemic 'stunned' myocardium by dimethylthiourea. Circulation. 1987;76:458–68.

84. Grieb P, Ryba MS, Debicki GS, Gordon-Krajcer W, Januszewski S, Chrapusta SJ. Changes in oxidative stress in the rat brain during post-cardiac arrest reperfusion, and the effect of treatment with the free radical scavenger idebenone. Resuscitation. 1998;39:107–13.
85. Taniguchi M, Uchinami M, Doi K, et al. Edaravone reduces ischemia-reperfusion injury mediators in rat liver. J Surg Res. 2007;137:69–74.
86. Watanabe T, Tahara M, Todo S. The novel antioxidant edaravone: from bench to bedside. Cardiovasc Ther. 2008;26:101–14.
87. Amaro S, Chamorro A. Translational stroke research of the combination of thrombolysis and antioxidant therapy. Stroke. 2011;42:1495–9.
88. Jain KK. Neuroprotection in cerebrovascular disease. Expert Opin Investig Drugs. 2000;9:695–711.
89. Zhang YE, Fu SZ, Li XQ, et al. PEP-1-SOD1 protects brain from ischemic insult following asphyxial cardiac arrest in rats. Resuscitation. 2011;82:1081–6.
90. Yamazaki K, Miwa S, Toyokuni S, et al. Effect of edaravone, a novel free radical scavenger, supplemented to cardioplegia on myocardial function after cardioplegic arrest: in vitro study of isolated rat heart. Heart Vessels. 2009;24:228–35.
91. Wiklund L, Sharma HS, Basu S. Circulatory arrest as a model for studies of global ischemic injury and neuroprotection. Ann N Y Acad Sci. 2005;1053:205–19.
92. Tang XN, Liu L, Yenari MA. Combination therapy with hypothermia for treatment of cerebral ischemia. J Neurotrauma. 2009;26:325–31.
93. Meybohm P, Gruenewald M, Albrecht M, et al. Hypothermia and postconditioning after cardiopulmonary resuscitation reduce cardiac dysfunction by modulating inflammation, apoptosis and remodeling. PLoS One. 2009;4:e7588.
94. Schwiebert C, Huhn R, Heinen A, et al. Postconditioning by xenon and hypothermia in the rat heart in vivo. Eur J Anaesthesiol. 2010;27: 734–9.
95. Schmid-Elsaesser R, Hungerhuber E, Zausinger S, Baethmann A, Reulen HJ. Combination drug therapy and mild hypothermia: a promising treatment strategy for reversible, focal cerebral ischemia. Stroke. 1999;30:1891–9.
96. Zausinger S, Scholler K, Plesnila N, Schmid-Elsaesser R. Combination drug therapy and mild hypothermia after transient focal cerebral ischemia in rats. Stroke. 2003;34:2246–51.
97. Scholler K, Zausinger S, Baethmann A, Schmid-Elsaesser R. Neuroprotection in ischemic stroke – combination drug therapy and mild hypothermia in a rat model of permanent focal cerebral ischemia. Brain Res. 2004;1023:272–8.
98. Aronowski J, Strong R, Shirzadi A, Grotta JC. Ethanol plus caffeine (caffeinol) for treatment of ischemic stroke: preclinical experience. Stroke. 2003;34:1246–51.
99. Martin-Schild S, Hallevi H, Shaltoni H, et al. Combined neuroprotective modalities coupled with thrombolysis in acute ischemic stroke: a pilot study of caffeinol and mild hypothermia. J Stroke Cerebrovasc Dis. 2009;18:86–96.
100. Nito C, Kamiya T, Ueda M, Arii T, Katayama Y. Mild hypothermia enhances the neuroprotective effects of FK506 and expands its therapeutic window following transient focal ischemia in rats. Brain Res. 2004;1008:179–85.
101. Dietrich WD, Busto R, Alonso O, Globus MY, Ginsberg MD. Intraischemic but not postischemic brain hypothermia protects chronically following global forebrain ischemia in rats. J Cereb Blood Flow Metab. 1993;13:541–9.
102. Green EJ, Dietrich WD, van Dijk F, et al. Protective effects of brain hypothermia on behavior and histopathology following global cerebral ischemia in rats. Brain Res. 1992;580:197–204.
103. Dietrich WD, Busto R, Bethea JR. Postischemic hypothermia and IL-10 treatment provide long-lasting neuroprotection of CA1 hippocampus following transient global ischemia in rats. Exp Neurol. 1999;158:444–50.
104. Meybohm P, Gruenewald M, Zacharowski KD, et al. Mild hypothermia alone or in combination with anesthetic post-conditioning reduces expression of inflammatory cytokines in the cerebral cortex of pigs after cardiopulmonary resuscitation. Crit Care. 2010;14:R21.
105. Holzer M. Targeted temperature management for comatose survivors of cardiac arrest. N Engl J Med. 2010;363:1256–64.
106. Holzer M, Bernard SA, Hachimi-Idrissi S, Roine RO, Sterz F, Mullner M. Hypothermia for neuroprotection after cardiac arrest: systematic review and individual patient data meta-analysis. Crit Care Med. 2005;33:414–8.
107. Abendschein DR, Tacker Jr WA, Babbs CF. Protection of ischemic myocardium by whole-body hypothermia after coronary artery occlusion in dogs. Am Heart J. 1978;96:772–80.
108. Ly HQ, Denault A, Dupuis J, et al. A pilot study: the Noninvasive Surface Cooling Thermoregulatory System for Mild Hypothermia Induction in Acute Myocardial Infarction (the NICAMI Study). Am Heart J. 2005;150:933.
109. Kandzari DE, Chu A, Brodie BR, et al. Feasibility of endovascular cooling as an adjunct to primary percutaneous coronary intervention (results of the LOWTEMP pilot study). Am J Cardiol. 2004;93: 636–9.
110. Stone GW, Dixon SR, Grines CL, et al. Predictors of infarct size after primary coronary angioplasty in acute myocardial infarction from pooled analysis from four contemporary trials. Am J Cardiol. 2007; 100:1370–5.
111. O'Neill WW, Dixon SR, Grines CL. The year in interventional cardiology. J Am Coll Cardiol. 2005;45:1117–34.
112. Tissier R, Chenoune M, Ghaleh B, Cohen MV, Downey JM, Berdeaux A. The small chill: mild

hypothermia for cardioprotection? Cardiovasc Res. 2010;88:406–14.
113. Busl KM, Greer DM. Hypoxic-ischemic brain injury: pathophysiology, neuropathology and mechanisms. NeuroRehabilitation. 2010;26:5–13.
114. Greer DM. Mechanisms of injury in hypoxic-ischemic encephalopathy: implications to therapy. Semin Neurol. 2006;26:373–9.
115. Hoesch RE, Koenig MA, Geocadin RG. Coma after global ischemic brain injury: pathophysiology and emerging therapies. Crit Care Clin. 2008;24:25–44. vii–viii.
116. Redmond JM, Gillinov AM, Zehr KJ, et al. Glutamate excitotoxicity: a mechanism of neurologic injury associated with hypothermic circulatory arrest. J Thorac Cardiovasc Surg. 1994;107:776–86. discussion 86–7.
117. Szydlowska K, Tymianski M. Calcium, ischemia and excitotoxicity. Cell Calcium. 2010;47:122–9.
118. Bokesch PM, Halpin DP, Ranger WR, et al. Immediate-early gene expression in ovine brain after hypothermic circulatory arrest: effects of aptiganel. Ann Thorac Surg. 1997;64:1082–7. discussion 8.
119. Nolan JP, Neumar RW, Adrie C, et al. Post-cardiac arrest syndrome: epidemiology, pathophysiology, treatment, and prognostication. A Scientific Statement from the International Liaison Committee on Resuscitation; the American Heart Association Emergency Cardiovascular Care Committee; the Council on Cardiovascular Surgery and Anesthesia; the Council on Cardiopulmonary, Perioperative, and Critical Care; the Council on Clinical Cardiology; the Council on Stroke. Resuscitation. 2008;79: 350–79.
120. Sterz F, Leonov Y, Safar P, et al. Multifocal cerebral blood flow by Xe-CT and global cerebral metabolism after prolonged cardiac arrest in dogs. Reperfusion with open-chest CPR or cardiopulmonary bypass. Resuscitation. 1992;24:27–47.
121. Ernster L. Biochemistry of reoxygenation injury. Crit Care Med. 1988;16:947–53.
122. McCullough JN, Zhang N, Reich DL, et al. Cerebral metabolic suppression during hypothermic circulatory arrest in humans. Ann Thorac Surg. 1999;67:1895–9. discussion 919–21.
123. D'Cruz BJ, Fertig KC, Filiano AJ, Hicks SD, DeFranco DB, Callaway CW. Hypothermic reperfusion after cardiac arrest augments brain-derived neurotrophic factor activation. J Cereb Blood Flow Metab. 2002;22:843–51.
124. Hachimi-Idrissi S, Van Hemelrijck A, Michotte A, et al. Postischemic mild hypothermia reduces neurotransmitter release and astroglial cell proliferation during reperfusion after asphyxial cardiac arrest in rats. Brain Res. 2004;1019:217–25.
125. Maier CM, Sun GH, Cheng D, Yenari MA, Chan PH, Steinberg GK. Effects of mild hypothermia on superoxide anion production, superoxide dismutase expression, and activity following transient focal cerebral ischemia. Neurobiol Dis. 2002;11:28–42.
126. Lei B, Tan X, Cai H, Xu Q, Guo Q. Effect of moderate hypothermia on lipid peroxidation in canine brain tissue after cardiac arrest and resuscitation. Stroke. 1994;25:147–52.
127. Eberspacher E, Werner C, Engelhard K, et al. Long-term effects of hypothermia on neuronal cell death and the concentration of apoptotic proteins after incomplete cerebral ischemia and reperfusion in rats. Acta Anaesthesiol Scand. 2005;49:477–87.
128. Webster CM, Kelly S, Koike MA, Chock VY, Giffard RG, Yenari MA. Inflammation and NFkappaB activation is decreased by hypothermia following global cerebral ischemia. Neurobiol Dis. 2009;33: 301–12.
129. Karibe H, Zarow GJ, Graham SH, Weinstein PR. Mild intraischemic hypothermia reduces postischemic hyperperfusion, delayed postischemic hypoperfusion, blood–brain barrier disruption, brain edema, and neuronal damage volume after temporary focal cerebral ischemia in rats. J Cereb Blood Flow Metab. 1994;14:620–7.
130. Sakurai A. Therapeutic hypothermia. Nihon Rinsho. 2011;69:642–7.
131. Hoehn T, Hansmann G, Buhrer C, et al. Therapeutic hypothermia in neonates. Review of current clinical data, ILCOR recommendations and suggestions for implementation in neonatal intensive care units. Resuscitation. 2008;78:7–12.
132. Wolfrum S, Radke PW, Pischon T, Willich SN, Schunkert H, Kurowski V. Mild therapeutic hypothermia after cardiac arrest – a nationwide survey on the implementation of the ILCOR guidelines in German intensive care units. Resuscitation. 2007; 72:207–13.
133. van der Worp HB, Sena ES, Donnan GA, Howells DW, Macleod MR. Hypothermia in animal models of acute ischaemic stroke: a systematic review and meta-analysis. Brain. 2007;130:3063–74.
134. Den Hertog HM, van der Worp HB, Tseng MC, Dippel DW. Cooling therapy for acute stroke. Cochrane Database Syst Rev. 2009: CD001247.
135. Hemmen TM, Lyden PD. Induced hypothermia for acute stroke. Stroke. 2007;38:794–9.
136. Dietrich WD, Alonso O, Busto R, et al. Posttraumatic cerebral ischemia after fluid percussion brain injury: an autoradiographic and histopathological study in rats. Neurosurgery. 1998;43:585–93. discussion 93–4.
137. Chesnut RM, Marshall SB, Piek J, Blunt BA, Klauber MR, Marshall LF. Early and late systemic hypotension as a frequent and fundamental source of cerebral ischemia following severe brain injury in the Traumatic Coma Data Bank. Acta Neurochir Suppl (Wien). 1993;59:121–5.
138. Matsushita Y, Bramlett HM, Alonso O, Dietrich WD. Posttraumatic hypothermia is neuroprotective in a model of traumatic brain injury complicated by a secondary hypoxic insult. Crit Care Med. 2001; 29:2060–6.
139. Muizelaar JP. Cerebral ischemia-reperfusion injury after severe head injury and its possible treatment

with polyethyleneglycol-superoxide dismutase. Ann Emerg Med. 1993;22:1014–21.
140. Miller JD, Bullock R, Graham DI, Chen MH, Teasdale GM. Ischemic brain damage in a model of acute subdural hematoma. Neurosurgery. 1990; 27:433–9.
141. Kuroda Y, Bullock R. Local cerebral blood flow mapping before and after removal of acute subdural hematoma in the rat. Neurosurgery. 1992;30: 687–91.
142. Burger R, Bendszus M, Vince GH, Solymosi L, Roosen K. Neurophysiological monitoring, magnetic resonance imaging, and histological assays confirm the beneficial effects of moderate hypothermia after epidural focal mass lesion development in rodents. Neurosurgery. 2004;54:701–11. discussion 11–2.
143. Clifton GL, Miller ER, Choi SC, et al. Lack of effect of induction of hypothermia after acute brain injury. N Engl J Med. 2001;344:556–63.
144. Clifton GL, Valadka A, Zygun D, et al. Very early hypothermia induction in patients with severe brain injury (the National Acute Brain Injury Study: Hypothermia II): a randomised trial. Lancet Neurol. 2011;10:131–9.
145. Farkas O, Povlishock JT. Cellular and subcellular change evoked by diffuse traumatic brain injury: a complex web of change extending far beyond focal damage. Prog Brain Res. 2007;161:43–59.
146. Jieyong B, Zhong W, Shiming Z, et al. Decompressive craniectomy and mild hypothermia reduces infarction size and counterregulates Bax and Bcl-2 expression after permanent focal ischemia in rats. Neurosurg Rev. 2006;29:168–72.
147. Liu MC, Akinyi L, Scharf D, et al. Ubiquitin C-terminal hydrolase-L1 as a biomarker for ischemic and traumatic brain injury in rats. Eur J Neurosci. 2010;31:722–32.
148. Papa L, Akinyi L, Liu MC, et al. Ubiquitin C-terminal hydrolase is a novel biomarker in humans for severe traumatic brain injury. Crit Care Med. 2010;38:138–44.
149. Okauchi M, Kawai N, Nakamura T, Kawanishi M, Nagao S. Effects of mild hypothermia and alkalizing agents on brain injuries in rats with acute subdural hematomas. J Neurotrauma. 2002;19:741–51.
150. Bederson JB, Pitts LH, Germano SM, Nishimura MC, Davis RL, Bartkowski HM. Evaluation of 2,3,5-triphenyltetrazolium chloride as a stain for detection and quantification of experimental cerebral infarction in rats. Stroke. 1986;17:1304–8.
151. Colbourne F, Corbett D. Delayed and prolonged post-ischemic hypothermia is neuroprotective in the gerbil. Brain Res. 1994;654:265–72.
152. Logue ES, McMichael MJ, Callaway CW. Comparison of the effects of hypothermia at 33 degrees C or 35 degrees C after cardiac arrest in rats. Acad Emerg Med. 2007;14:293–300.

4 Cardiac Arrest: Who Should Be Cooled?

Sanjeev U. Nair and Justin B. Lundbye

Introduction

Approximately 300,000 out-of-hospital and 20,000 in-hospital cardiac arrests occur annually in the United States [1], and an estimated 92–189 out-of-hospital cardiac arrests per 100,000 population occur annually in industrialized nations [2, 3]. The use of therapeutic hypothermia (TH) in cardiac arrest survivors has been advocated in order to mitigate the neurologic injury that transpires as a result of hypoxia and reperfusion [4]. The precise mechanisms by which mild hypothermia is beneficial in these patients is unclear at present but the supposition is that mild hypothermia modifies various chemical and cellular pathways that cause necrosis and apoptosis of neurons [4] (see Chap. 2). Moreover, it has beneficial effects on various other organ systems which bear the brunt of the post-cardiac arrest state [5]. With the rising popularity of mild therapeutic hypothermia (32–34°C) in cardiac arrest patients, there is a continuing need to appropriately select patients who will benefit from its use. This chapter attempts to interpret the available information and provide direction on selecting appropriate adult cardiac arrest patients who may benefit from the use of therapeutic hypothermia (TH).

S.U. Nair, MBBS, M.D., FACP(✉)
J.B. Lundbye, M.D., FACC
Division of Cardiology,
Henry Low Heart Center, Hartford Hospital,
Hartford, CT, USA

University of Connecticut School of Medicine,
Farmington, CT, USA
e-mail: jlundbye@thocc.org; doc_nsu@rediffmail.com

Published Studies

The Evidence for Use of TH in Cardiac Arrest Due to Shockable Rhythms (Ventricular Fibrillation or Pulseless Ventricular Tachycardia) (Table 4.1)

Initial case reports followed by small prospective studies which used historical controls at single centers showed the promise of mild hypothermia in out-of-hospital ventricular fibrillation survivors [6–14]. Following these, the HACA study group [15] performed a multicenter randomized control trial in centers across Europe on 275 adult patients who sustained out-of-hospital cardiac arrest due to ventricular fibrillation. Of the study cohort, 137 patients received hypothermia to 32–34°C for 24 h with an external cooling device. Following 24 h of cooling, they were passively rewarmed over 8 h. The study resulted in 55% of the hypothermia group having a significantly better neurologic outcome as compared to 39% in the normothermia group (P=0.009). Moreover, the 6-month mortality was 41% in the hypothermia group in comparison to 55% in the normothermia group (P=0.02). Although this study ended prematurely due to lack of funds, it demonstrated that therapeutic hypothermia in patients successfully resuscitated

J.B. Lundbye (ed.), *Therapeutic Hypothermia After Cardiac Arrest*,
DOI 10.1007/978-1-4471-2951-6_4, © Springer-Verlag London 2012

Table 4.1 Published studies on TH and outcomes in cardiac arrest survivors

Trial	Study design	Number of study patients	Cooling method	Rhythm	Survival (TH vs. control)	Neurologic outcome (TH vs. control)
Bernard et al. [7]	Historical control	44	External	All	55% vs. 23%, P<0.05	50% vs. 14%,P<0.05
Yanagawa et al. [6]	Historical control	28	External	All	54% vs. 33%, P <0.05	23% vs. 7%, P<0.05
Bernard et al. [16]	Pseuo-randomized controlled	77	External	VF	49% vs. 32%, P=0.145	48% vs. 26%, P=0.046
The HACA study group [15]	Randomized control	275	External	VF/VT	59% vs. 45%, P=0.02	55% vs. 39%, P=0.009
Oddo et al. [23]	Historical control	109	External	All	VF:60% vs. 44%, P=0.28	VF:56% vs. 26%, P=0.004
					PEA/asystole: 17% vs. 9%	PEA/asystole: 17% vs. 0%
Busch et al. [38]	Historical control	61	External	All	59% vs. 32%, P=0.05	41% vs. 26%, P=0.21
Knafeij et al. [29]	Historical control	72	External	STEMI with VF	75% vs. 14%, P=0.0014	55% vs. 16%, P=0.001
Bellard et al. [39]	Historical control	68	External	VF	56% vs. 36%, P=0.04	72% vs. 46%, P=0.02
Sunde et al. [28]	Historical control	119	Internal or external	All	56% vs. 31%, P =0.007	56% vs. 26%, P<0.001
Storm et al. [25]	Historical control	126	External	All	71% vs. 58%, P=0.19	62% vs. 23%, P<0.001
Don et al. [22]	Historical control	491	External	All	VF/VT: 54% vs. 39%, P=0.04	VF/VT: 35% vs. 15%, P<0.01
					PEA/asystole: 21% vs. 19%, P=0.65	PEA/asystole: 12% vs. 9%, P=0.44
Bro-Jeppesen et al. [40]	Historical control	156	External	All	VF/VT: 67% vs. 68%, P =0.79	VF/VT: 97% vs. 71%, P=0.003
Castrejon et al. [41]	Historical control	69	External	VF/VT	56% vs. 39%, P =0.17	44% vs. 18%, P=0.029
Dumas et al. [24]	Historical control	1,145	External	All	VF/VT:44% vs. 29%, P<0.001	Analyses not performed
					PEA/asystole: 15% vs. 17%, P=0.48	
Lundbye et al. [18]	Historical control	100	External + internal	PEA/asystole	39% vs. 19%, P=0.03	29% vs. 13%, P=0.02
Testori et al. [19]	Historical control	374	External + internal	PEA/asystole	35% vs. 23%, P=0.024	39% vs. 25%, P=0.025

PEA pulseless electrical activity, *STEMI* ST- elevation myocardial infarction, *TH* therapeutic hypothermia, *VF* ventricular fibrillation, *VT* ventricular tachycardia from cardiac arrest due to a shockable rhythm resulted in improved neurological outcome and survival. Bernard et al. [16] in a multicenter pseudo-randomized study performed across Australia, demonstrated the efficacy of therapeutic hypothermia in 77 adult patients who were successfully resuscitated after an out-of-hospital cardiac arrest due to ventricular fibrillation. Of the study cohort, 43 patients were given TH using ice packs as compared to 34 patients who had normothermia. Forty nine percent of the patients who underwent hypothermia as compared to twenty six percent in the normothermia group were discharged to home or a rehabilitation facility with better neurologic recovery (P=0.046).

Since the publication of these two landmark trials, there have been a number of observational and retrospective studies on the use of TH especially in VF/pulseless VT. Some of the more relevant trials pertaining to the use of TH in patients with cardiac arrest due to ventricular fibrillation or pulseless ventricular tachycardia are summarized in Table 4.1.

The Evidence for Use of TH in Cardiac Arrest Due to Non-shockable Rhythms (Pulseless Electrical Activity and Asystole) (Tables 4.1 and 4.2)

To date no randomized control trials have addressed the efficacy of TH in cardiac arrest patients successfully resuscitated from pulseless electrical activity or asystole. However, a multitude of observational and retrospective studies have attempted to address this aspect. In an observational study by Arrich et al. [17] where cooling was achieved mostly via an endovascular device on 197 cardiac arrest patients with pulseless electrical activity or asystole, therapeutic hypothermia showed significant mortality benefit, although there was no effect on neurologic outcome. In two recent retrospective studies by Lundbye et al. [18] and Testori et al. [19], the use of TH in patients with non-shockable rhythms (PEA and asystole) was associated with improved neurologic and survival outcomes. Lundbye et al. performed a retrospective study on 100 cardiac arrest patients successfully resuscitated from either PEA or asystole. Fifteen (29%) of the 52 patients who underwent TH had good neurologic outcome as compared to 5 (10%) of the 43 patients who were historical controls (P=0.021). The adjusted odds ratio for a good neurologic outcome and survival at hospital discharge with TH were 4.35 (95% Confidence Interval 1.10–17.24, P=0.004) and 5.65 (95% Confidence Interval 1.66–19.23, P=0.006) respectively. Testori et al. compared 135 patients who were successfully resuscitated from either PEA or asystole and who underwent TH with 239 similar patients who did not undergo TH. A total of 47 patients (35%) who underwent TH as compared to 55 patients (23%) in the control group had a significantly better neurologic outcome with an adjusted odds ratio of 1.84 (95% Confidence Interval 1.08–3.13, P=0.024). Similarly 180 patients (75%) in the hypothermia group as compared to 82 patients (61%) in the control group had a significantly better 6-month survival outcome with an adjusted odds ratio of death of 0.56 (95%

Table 4.2 Systematic review/meta-analysis on TH and outcomes

Author	Types of study included	Number of patients	Neurologic outcome with TH	Survival outcome with TH
Kim et al. [20]	2 RCT and 12 NRCT (non-shockable rhythm)	1,336	RCT's: no analyses done	RCT's: RR for death=0.85 (95% CI: 0.65–1.11)
			NRCT's: RR for poor outcome=0.95 (95% CI: 0.90–1.01)	NRCT's: RR for death=0.84 (95% CI: 0.78–0.92)
Arrich et al. [17]	4 RCT and 1 abstract (all rhythms)	481	RR for good outcome=1.55 (95% CI:1.22–1.96)	RR for good outcome=1.35 (95% CI;1.10–1.65)
Nielsen et al. [21]	5 RCT (all rhythms)	478	RR for poor outcome = 0.78 (95% CI: 0.64–0.95)	RR for death=0.84 (95% CI: 0.70–1.01)

NRCT non-randomized control trial, *RCT* randomized control trial, *RR* relative risk, *TH* therapeutic hypothermia

Confidence Interval 0.34–0.93, P=0.025). In a recently published meta-analysis by Kim et al. [20] which included 14 studies on the efficacy of TH in cardiac arrest survivors there was a significant benefit of TH on survival outcome in cardiac arrest survivors of non-shockable rhythms with a pooled RR of 0.84 (95% Confidence Interval 0.78–0.92, $I^2=0\%$). Data on studies on the use of TH in patients with cardiac arrest due to pulseless electrical activity and asystole is summarized in Table 4.2.

Published Evidence Showing Neutral Benefit of TH in Cardiac Arrest Survivors (Tables 4.1 and 4.2)

Nielsen et al. [21] in a recent meta-analysis of five randomized trials of TH in cardiac arrest survivors found no benefit on the use of TH in improving neurologic or survival outcomes. They reported that the evidence was inconclusive and thus there is clinical equipoise in its use in such patients.

Retrospective studies performed by Don et al. [22] and Oddo et al. [23], on out-of-hospital cardiac arrest patients failed to demonstrate a significant improvement in survival or neurologic outcome in the subgroup of patients with non-shockable rhythms who received therapeutic hypothermia as compared to historic controls. The former study by Don et al. included 313 cardiac arrest survivors of non-shockable rhythms. In this subgroup, 121 patients who underwent TH did not show any significant benefit in either neurologic or survival outcome as compared to 191 historical control patients. This lack of benefit in the subgroup of patients with non-shockable rhythms is possibly due to the multiple factors which include the use of surface cooling which may be less effective in achieving target temperature when compared with intravascular cooling and that the time to ROSC of study patients was prolonged leading to a delay in time to achieve target temperature. The study performed by Oddo et al. on a cohort of 23 patients with non-shockable rhythms was perhaps underpowered to draw any significant conclusions. In an observational study performed by Dumas et al. [24] on out-of-hospital cardiac arrest patients, 437 patients had non-shockable rhythms. Out of these, 261 patients (60%) underwent therapeutic hypothermia with external cooling as compared to 176 patients (40%) who were not cooled. Their study showed no benefit of hypothermia therapy on neurologic outcome in patients with non-shockable rhythms. There were several limitations to this study, particularly the delay to ROSC was substantial in the hypothermia arm and also the time to achieve target temperature was almost 9 h from initiation of TH. The authors concluded that the lack of benefit of TH in their study is perhaps a result of an inadequate "dose" of hypothermia in terms of degree and duration commensurate with the circulatory status of their patients. Moreover, they felt that patients with non-shockable rhythms were more likely to have a non-cardiac cause for cardiac arrest placing TH at a higher risk-benefit ratio in these patients. More recently, Storm et al. [25] performed an observational study on 175 cardiac arrest survivors which included 87 patients who underwent TH as compared to 88 historical control patients. Although there was a trend towards benefit in improving neurologic outcome while using TH in cardiac arrest survivors of non-shockable rhythms, the results were not statistically significant. The authors conclude that the higher Acute Physiology and Chronic Health Evaluation (APACHE) scores of the hypothermia group as compared to the control group may have contributed to this finding.

What the Guidelines Say

Based on published literature on the efficacy of TH in cardiac arrest survivors, the International Liaison Committee on Resuscitation (ILCOR) issued a special report in 2003 recommending that "Unconscious adult patients with spontaneous circulation after out-of-hospital cardiac arrest should be cooled to 32–34°C for 12–24 h when the initial rhythm was ventricular fibrillation (VF) (Class IIa). Such cooling may also be beneficial for other rhythms or in-hospital cardiac arrest (Class IIb)" [26].

The guidelines on post-cardiac arrest care have been recently updated by the American Heart Association (AHA) and the recommendations are [27]:

Table 4.3 Indications and contraindications for TH in adult comatose cardiac arrest survivors

Adult cardiac arrest survivors in whom TH is indicated	Absolute or relative contraindications to TH in adult cardiac arrest survivors
Patients with out-of hospital ventricular fibrillation/pulseless ventricular tachycardia (Class I, LOE B)	Core body temperature <30°C on admission
Patients with out-of hospital PEA/asystole (Class IIb, LOE B)	Pregnancy
Patients with in-hospital cardiac arrest (Class IIb, LOE B)	Terminally ill
	DNR status
	Severe sepsis/septic shock
	Severe bleeding disorder
	CPC 3–4 or GCS ≤8 prior to cardiac arrest
	Shock not responsive to vasopressor and/or mechanical support
	Downtime >30 min or unwitnessed asystole of unknown duration
	Elapse of greater than 6 h after ROSC
	Intracranial hemorrhage

CPC Cerebral Performance Scale, *DNR* do not resuscitate, *GCS* Glasgow Coma Scale, *LOE* level of evidence, *TH* therapeutic hypothermia, *ROSC* return of spontaneous circulation

1. Comatose (i.e. lack of meaningful response to verbal commands) adult patients with ROSC after out-of-hospital VF cardiac arrest should be cooled to 32–34°C (89.6–93.2°F) for 12–24 h (Class I, LOE B).
2. Induced hypothermia also may be considered for comatose adult patients with ROSC after in-hospital cardiac arrest of any initial rhythm or after out-of-hospital cardiac arrest with an initial rhythm of pulseless electric activity or asystole (Class IIb, LOE B).

Cardiac Arrest Patients Least Likely to Benefit from TH

Most contraindications for the use of TH in cardiac arrest survivors are relative and are expected to continually change as emerging data on this therapy gets published (Table 4.3). TH is relatively contraindicated in presence of severe sepsis and severe active bleeding, as there is an increased risk of both infection and bleeding at low body temperatures. Therapeutic hypothermia is not useful in the presence of advanced malignancy and severe chronic disease with poor life expectancy. Therapeutic hypothermia is presently not recommended in patients with suspected or confirmed cerebrovascular accident leading to cardiac arrest. TH is not a recommended therapy in patients with unwitnessed asystole when the duration of cardiac arrest cannot be estimated. It is not recommended in patients with a pre-cardiac arrest Cerebral Performance Category of 3–4 or a Glasgow Coma Scale of ≤8. It is also not recommended in those patients in whom the CPR duration till ROSC is greater than 30 min or if more than 6 h have elapsed after successful CPR and ROSC. Presently TH is not recommended in states of hemodynamic shock which is not responsive to vasopressor or mechanical support. It remains contraindicated in pregnancy since no safety data of its use in these patients is available. Patients who have elected to not have resuscitation are not candidates for TH. Cardiac arrest survivors who are already hypothermic (T° <30°C) on admission may not need to have TH.

Evolving Issues with TH in Subgroups of Cardiac Arrest Survivors

Use with Percutaneous Coronary Intervention (PCI)

Recent studies with historical controls have shown that it is safe and feasible to use primary PCI with TH in cardiac arrest patients [28–30]. However, further studies should address the role of this combined treatment in reducing infarct size and cardiac reperfusion injury as well as its effect on neurologic and survival outcomes (see Chap. 10). Moreover, the effect of hypothermia on the efficacy of anti-platelet medications in patients who undergo PCI is presently not clear [31].

Use in Cardiogenic Shock

Studies that have addressed TH in cardiac arrest survivors with cardiogenic shock demonstrate promising results [32–34]. Although questions regarding the degree and duration of cooling in these patients e.g. the need for a higher "dose" of hypothermia in presence of cardiogenic shock, are still unanswered (see Chap. 10).

Use in Non-shockable Rhythms

As noted earlier there remains a continuing debate on whether TH is as useful in patients with non-shockable rhythms as it is in patients with shockable rhythms. Although the neuropathophysiologic changes that take place post-cardiac arrest may be independent of the type of rhythm, patients with non-shockable rhythms are likely to be more heterogeneous with regards to co-morbidities and the etiology of cardiac arrest as compared to those with shockable rhythms. Thus there is a need for clinical tools that can help with selection of patients with non-shockable rhythms who are most likely to benefit from TH [35].

Use in In-Hospital Cardiac Arrest

There may be a reduced efficacy of TH in patients with in-hospital cardiac arrest since these patients are more likely to be "sicker", have non-shockable rhythms and have cardiac arrest secondary to a non-cardiac cause as compared to patients with out-of hospital cardiac arrest. Most studies demonstrating the benefit of TH in cardiac arrest survivors have either exclusively looked at out-of hospital cardiac arrests or have consisted of small numbers of in-hospital cardiac arrest patients [15, 16, 36, 37]. Thus the role of TH in patients successfully resuscitated after in-hospital cardiac arrest needs further investigation.

At this time there are no randomized controlled trials planned to address these specific populations and we will have to rely on observational and retrospective studies to continue to find the answers.

Conclusions

Historically, cardiac arrest survivors have had poor neurologic and long-term survival outcomes. Based on emerging evidence of its efficacy in improving neurologic and survival outcomes, Therapeutic Hypothermia (TH) has become standard of care in select cardiac arrest survivors. Its role in specific populations of cardiac arrest survivors, especially those with non-shockable rhythms as well as in those who arrested in-hospital, remains unclear. Further randomized controlled trials are desperately needed to address these issues.

References

1. Roger VL, Go AS, Lloyd-Jones DM, Adams RJ, Berry JD, Brown TM, Carnethon MR, Dai S, de Simone G, Ford ES, Fox CS, Fullerton HJ, Gillespie C, Greenlund KJ, Hailpern SM, Heit JA, Ho PM, Howard VJ, Kissela BM, Kittner SJ, Lackland DT, Lichtman JH, Lisabeth LD, Makuc DM, Marcus GM, Marelli A, Matchar DB, McDermott MM, Meigs JB, Moy CS, Mozaffarian D, Mussolino ME, Nichol G, Paynter NP, Rosamond WD, Sorlie PD, Stafford RS, Turan TN, Turner MB, Wong ND, Wylie-Rosett J. Heart disease and stroke statistics – 2011 update: a report from the American Heart Association. Circulation. 2011;123(4):e18–209.
2. Straus SM, Bleumink GS, Dieleman JP, van der LJ, Stricker BH, Sturkenboom MC. The incidence of sudden cardiac death in the general population. J Clin Epidemiol. 2004;57(1):98–102.
3. Nichol G, Thomas E, Callaway CW, Hedges J, Powell JL, Aufderheide TP, Rea T, Lowe R, Brown T, Dreyer J, Davis D, Idris A, Stiell I. Regional variation in out-of-hospital cardiac arrest incidence and outcome. JAMA. 2008;300(12):1423–31.
4. Gonzalez-Ibarra FP, Varon J, Lopez-Meza EG. Therapeutic hypothermia: critical review of the molecular mechanisms of action. Front Neurol. 2011;2:4.

5. Nolan JP, Neumar RW, Adrie C, Aibiki M, Berg RA, Bottiger BW, Callaway C, Clark RS, Geocadin RG, Jauch EC, Kern KB, Laurent I, Longstreth WT, Merchant RM, Morley P, Morrison LJ, Nadkarni V, Peberdy MA, Rivers EP, Rodriguez-Nunez A, Sellke FW, Spaulding C, Sunde K, Hoek TV. Post-cardiac arrest syndrome: epidemiology, pathophysiology, treatment, and prognostication. A Scientific Statement from the International Liaison Committee on Resuscitation; the American Heart Association Emergency Cardiovascular Care Committee; the Council on Cardiovascular Surgery and Anesthesia; the Council on Cardiopulmonary, Perioperative, and Critical Care; the Council on Clinical Cardiology; the Council on Stroke. Resuscitation. 2008;79(3):350–79.
6. Yanagawa Y, Ishihara S, Norio H, Takino M, Kawakami M, Takasu A, Okamoto K, Kaneko N, Terai C, Okada Y. Preliminary clinical outcome study of mild resuscitative hypothermia after out-of-hospital cardiopulmonary arrest. Resuscitation. 1998;39(1–2):61–6.
7. Bernard SA, Jones BM, Horne MK. Clinical trial of induced hypothermia in comatose survivors of out-of-hospital cardiac arrest. Ann Emerg Med. 1997;30(2):146–53.
8. Benson DW, Williams Jr GR, Spencer FC, Yates AJ. The use of hypothermia after cardiac arrest. Anesth Analg. 1959;38:423–8.
9. Williams Jr GR, Spencer FC. The clinical use of hypothermia following cardiac arrest. Ann Surg. 1958;148(3):462–8.
10. Sanada T, Ueki M, Tokudome M, Okamura T, Nishiki S, Niimura A, Yabuki S, Watanabe Y. Recovery from out-of-hospital cardiac arrest after mild hypothermia: report of two cases. Masui. 1998;47(6):742–5.
11. Nagao K, Hayashi N, Kanmatsuse K, Arima K, Ohtsuki J, Kikushima K, Watanabe I. Cardiopulmonary cerebral resuscitation using emergency cardiopulmonary bypass, coronary reperfusion therapy and mild hypothermia in patients with cardiac arrest outside the hospital. J Am Coll Cardiol. 2000;36(3):776–83.
12. Zeiner A, Holzer M, Sterz F, Behringer W, Schorkhuber W, Mullner M, Frass M, Siostrzonek P, Ratheiser K, Kaff A, Laggner AN. Mild resuscitative hypothermia to improve neurological outcome after cardiac arrest. A clinical feasibility trial. Hypothermia After Cardiac Arrest (HACA) Study Group. Stroke. 2000;31(1):86–94.
13. Felberg RA, Krieger DW, Chuang R, Persse DE, Burgin WS, Hickenbottom SL, Morgenstern LB, Rosales O, Grotta JC. Hypothermia after cardiac arrest: feasibility and safety of an external cooling protocol. Circulation. 2001;104(15):1799–804.
14. Hachimi-Idrissi S, Corne L, Ebinger G, Michotte Y, Huyghens L. Mild hypothermia induced by a helmet device: a clinical feasibility study. Resuscitation. 2001;51(3):275–81.
15. Hypothermia after Cardiac Arrest Study Group. Mild therapeutic hypothermia to improve the neurologic outcome after cardiac arrest. N Engl J Med. 2002;346(8):549–56.
16. Bernard SA, Gray TW, Buist MD, Jones BM, Silvester W, Gutteridge G, Smith K. Treatment of comatose survivors of out-of-hospital cardiac arrest with induced hypothermia. N Engl J Med. 2002;346(8):557–63.
17. Arrich J, Holzer M, Herkner H, Mullner M. Cochrane corner: hypothermia for neuroprotection in adults after cardiopulmonary resuscitation. Anesth Analg. 2010;110(4):1239.
18. Lundbye JB, Rai M, Ramu B, Hosseini-Khalili A, Li D, Slim HB, Bhavnani SP, Nair SU, Kluger J. Therapeutic hypothermia is associated with improved neurologic outcome and survival in cardiac arrest survivors of non-shockable rhythms. Resuscitation. 2012;83(2):202–7.
19. Testori C, Sterz F, Behringer W, Haugk M, Uray T, Zeiner A, Janata A, Arrich J, Holzer M, Losert H. Mild therapeutic hypothermia is associated with favourable outcome in patients after cardiac arrest with non-shockable rhythms. Resuscitation. 2011;82(9):1162–7.
20. Kim YM, Yim HW, Jeong SH, Klem ML, Callaway CW. Does therapeutic hypothermia benefit adult cardiac arrest patients presenting with non-shockable initial rhythms?: A systematic review and meta-analysis of randomized and non-randomized studies. Resuscitation. 2012;83(2):188–96.
21. Nielsen N, Hovdenes J, Nilsson F, Rubertsson S, Stammet P, Sunde K, Valsson F, Wanscher M, Friberg H. Outcome, timing and adverse events in therapeutic hypothermia after out-of-hospital cardiac arrest. Acta Anaesthesiol Scand. 2009;53(7):926–34.
22. Don CW, Longstreth Jr WT, Maynard C, Olsufka M, Nichol G, Ray T, Kupchik N, Deem S, Copass MK, Cobb LA, Kim F. Active surface cooling protocol to induce mild therapeutic hypothermia after out-of-hospital cardiac arrest: a retrospective before-and-after comparison in a single hospital. Crit Care Med. 2009;37(12):3062–9.
23. Oddo M, Ribordy V, Feihl F, Rossetti AO, Schaller MD, Chiolero R, Liaudet L. Early predictors of outcome in comatose survivors of ventricular fibrillation and non-ventricular fibrillation cardiac arrest treated with hypothermia: a prospective study. Crit Care Med. 2008;36(8):2296–301.
24. Dumas F, Grimaldi D, Zuber B, Fichet J, Charpentier J, Pene F, Vivien B, Varenne O, Carli P, Jouven X, Empana JP, Cariou A. Is hypothermia after cardiac arrest effective in both shockable and nonshockable patients?: insights from a large registry. Circulation. 2011;123(8):877–86.
25. Storm C, Steffen I, Schefold JC, Krueger A, Oppert M, Jorres A, Hasper D. Mild therapeutic hypothermia shortens intensive care unit stay of survivors after out-of-hospital cardiac arrest compared to historical controls. Crit Care. 2008;12(3):R78.
26. Nolan JP, Morley PT, Hoek TL, Hickey RW. Therapeutic hypothermia after cardiac arrest. An advisory statement by the Advancement Life support Task Force of the International Liaison committee on Resuscitation. Resuscitation. 2003;57(3):231–5.

27. Peberdy MA, Callaway CW, Neumar RW, Geocadin RG, Zimmerman JL, Donnino M, Gabrielli A, Silvers SM, Zaritsky AL, Merchant R, Vanden Hoek TL, Kronick SL. Part 9: post-cardiac arrest care: 2010 American Heart Association Guidelines for Cardiopulmonary Resuscitation and Emergency Cardiovascular Care. Circulation. 2010;122(18 Suppl 3): S768–86.
28. Sunde K, Pytte M, Jacobsen D, Mangschau A, Jensen LP, Smedsrud C, Draegni T, Steen PA. Implementation of a standardised treatment protocol for post resuscitation care after out-of-hospital cardiac arrest. Resuscitation. 2007;73(1):29–39.
29. Knafelj R, Radsel P, Ploj T, Noc M. Primary percutaneous coronary intervention and mild induced hypothermia in comatose survivors of ventricular fibrillation with ST-elevation acute myocardial infarction. Resuscitation. 2007;74(2):227–34.
30. Wolfrum S, Pierau C, Radke PW, Schunkert H, Kurowski V. Mild therapeutic hypothermia in patients after out-of-hospital cardiac arrest due to acute ST-segment elevation myocardial infarction undergoing immediate percutaneous coronary intervention. Crit Care Med. 2008;36(6):1780–6.
31. Bjelland TW, Hjertner O, Klepstad P, Kaisen K, Dale O, Haugen BO. Antiplatelet effect of clopidogrel is reduced in patients treated with therapeutic hypothermia after cardiac arrest. Resuscitation. 2010;81(12):1627–31.
32. Hovdenes J, Laake JH, Aaberge L, Haugaa H, Bugge JF. Therapeutic hypothermia after out-of-hospital cardiac arrest: experiences with patients treated with percutaneous coronary intervention and cardiogenic shock. Acta Anaesthesiol Scand. 2007;51(2):137–42.
33. Oddo M, Schaller MD, Feihl F, Ribordy V, Liaudet L. From evidence to clinical practice: effective implementation of therapeutic hypothermia to improve patient outcome after cardiac arrest. Crit Care Med. 2006;34(7):1865–73.
34. Skulec R, Kovarnik T, Dostalova G, Kolar J, Linhart A. Induction of mild hypothermia in cardiac arrest survivors presenting with cardiogenic shock syndrome. Acta Anaesthesiol Scand. 2008;52(2):188–94.
35. Bhavnani SP, Rai M, Chua NY, Engles D, Kluger J, Lundbye JB. Risk assessment model for survival with good neurologic recovery after cardiac arrest and treatment with therapeutic hypothermia. The Hartford hypothermia risk score. J Am Coll Cardiol. 2011; 57: 2019.
36. Arrich J. Clinical application of mild therapeutic hypothermia after cardiac arrest. Crit Care Med. 2007;35(4):1041–7.
37. Holzer M, Mullner M, Sterz F, Robak O, Kliegel A, Losert H, Sodeck G, Uray T, Zeiner A, Laggner AN. Efficacy and safety of endovascular cooling after cardiac arrest: cohort study and Bayesian approach. Stroke. 2006;37(7):1792–7.
38. Busch M, Soreide E, Lossius HM, Lexow K, Dickstein K. Rapid implementation of therapeutic hypothermia in comatose out-of-hospital cardiac arrest survivors. Acta Anaesthesiol Scand. 2006;50(10):1277–83.
39. Belliard G, Catez E, Charron C, Caille V, Aegerter P, Dubourg O, Jardin F, Vieillard-Baron A. Efficacy of therapeutic hypothermia after out-of-hospital cardiac arrest due to ventricular fibrillation. Resuscitation. 2007;75(2):252–9.
40. Bro-Jeppesen J, Kjaergaard J, Horsted TI, Wanscher MC, Nielsen SL, Rasmussen LS, Hassager C. The impact of therapeutic hypothermia on neurological function and quality of life after cardiac arrest. Resuscitation. 2009;80(2):171–6.
41. Castrejon S, Cortes M, Salto ML, Benittez LC, Rubio R, Juarez M, de Lopez SE, Bueno H, Sanchez PL, Fernandez AF. Improved prognosis after using mild hypothermia to treat cardiorespiratory arrest due to a cardiac cause: comparison with a control group. Rev Esp Cardiol. 2009;62(7):733–41.

Hypothermia: How to Cool

5

Matthew W. Parker and Justin B. Lundbye

Introduction

Prompt and expert institution of therapeutic hypothermia is key to optimizing neurologic outcomes after cardiac arrest. In general, therapeutic hypothermia entails lowering the cardiac arrest survivor's body temperature by any combination of infusing cold saline, applying ice packs, applying a cold-air mattress or cold-water circulating pads to the body, or inserting intravascular catheters that circulate cold water. Consideration must be given to temperature monitoring as well as patient comfort, particularly as regards shivering.

At the same time, cardiac arrest survivors are critically ill in the post-arrest period, a condition referred to as the post-cardiac arrest syndrome [1]. Therefore, application of therapeutic hypothermia must be integrated within the overall care of critically ill patients, who often require multiple diagnostic and therapeutic procedures promptly following a cardiac arrest. The techniques for applying therapeutic hypothermia must therefore enable rapid, effective temperature control without interfering with other life-saving therapies. Several commercial systems are available, each with unique abilities and limitations in this regard, and the local critical care team must be familiar with the application and pitfalls of the method used in their institution. This chapter will discuss the issues of inducing, maintaining, and reversing therapeutic hypothermia after cardiac arrest, and briefly summarize adjunctive therapies that may be useful when applying therapeutic hypothermia. Finally, the practice at the authors' institution will be presented as an example of how therapeutic hypothermia might be implemented.

M.W. Parker, M.D. (✉) • J.B. Lundbye, M.D., FACC
Division of Cardiology, Henry Low Heart Center,
Hartford Hospital, Department of Medicine,
Henry Low Heart Center 80 Seymour Street,
Hartford, CT 06102, USA

University of Connecticut School of Medicine,
Department of Medicine, Farmington, CT, USA
e-mail: mwparker@harthosp.org;
jlundby@harthosp.org

Induction

Induction of therapeutic hypothermia refers to initial cooling of the body's core temperature. This initial cooling requires a large transfer of heat energy from the body and should begin as expeditiously as possible once the decision is made to pursue therapeutic hypothermia. Animal studies have shown that a delay of as little as 15 min after return of circulation before the onset of cooling could attenuate the benefit of hypothermia after an induced VF arrest [2] and that a 24-h period of hypothermia after cardiac arrest in dogs produced the best neurologic recovery when begun 1 h after return of spontaneous circulation but could still be beneficial if started 4 h after resuscitation [3]. Observational data in humans have demonstrated that earlier time to target temperature is associated with higher rates of neurologic recovery. In a series of 49 patients reported

J.B. Lundbye (ed.), *Therapeutic Hypothermia After Cardiac Arrest*,
DOI 10.1007/978-1-4471-2951-6_5, © Springer-Verlag London 2012

by Wolff and colleagues, the chances of a favorable neurologic outcome declined by almost a third with every hour delay in achieving mild therapeutic hypothermia [4]. Multiplying this odds ratio over several hours yields a significant drop-off in benefit, consistent with the animal models.

Mild hypothermia, or a core temperature of 32–34°C, was associated with improved neurological outcomes among survivors of cardiac arrest due to ventricular fibrillation or pulseless ventricular tachycardia in interventional trials in Europe and Australia [5, 6]. This same temperature range should therefore be used clinically. Core body temperature refers to the internal body temperature, as measured with a probe placed in the esophagus or a central vein. Rectal or urinary bladder temperature measurements may be more easily obtained, although these do not correlate as well with brain temperature [7]. Tympanic temperature is not sufficiently accurate as a measure of therapeutic hypothermia but may be used as a screening tool: patients with tympanic temperatures <30°C are not likely to benefit from further lowering of the body temperature and have been excluded from the major trials of therapeutic hypothermia after cardiac arrest.

In a critically ill patient following a cardiac arrest, multiple competing demands such as primary percutaneous intervention for acute coronary syndromes and transport to tertiary care center for most patients may prevent immediate induction of therapeutic hypothermia. However, the method used for induction does not have to be the same as that ultimately used for maintenance, and so cooling can begin even as other life-saving therapies are undertaken. This also means that community hospitals that will transfer patients to referral centers for intensive care, cooling can start with methods available locally prior to transfer and then be continued at in the intensive care unit.

Mild therapeutic hypothermia may be induced by rapid, large-volume (30 ml/kg) infusion of ice-cold (4°C) saline as long as pulmonary edema is not present. In a study of 22 comatose survivors of cardiac arrest, this strategy lowered mean core temperature from 35.5°C to 33.8°C in 30 min with no adverse effects [8]. This has the distinct advantage that it requires only cold saline and intravenous access to administer. Pulmonary edema is obviously a concern and this approach is only useful for induction, not maintenance, of hypothermia because of the attendant intravascular volume loading.

Ice packs may be applied around the head, neck, torso, and limbs; this was the principle method of cooling used in the Australian trial but may be less effective in patients with larger body mass. One external commercial system (ThermoSuit, LifeRecovery Systems, Kinnelon, NJ) has been developed specifically for induction of hypothermia. The patient is placed in the device, which irrigates the skin with cold water, rapidly cooling the body. Although this approach would not be feasible for maintenance use over a period of days, it may be well-suited for induction of hypothermia in emergency rooms prior to transfer to the intensive care unit.

Effective induction of mild therapeutic hypothermia was recently demonstrated using an intranasal device with an evaporative coolant in a European study [9]. Two hundred cardiac arrest survivors were randomized to pre-hospital intranasal cooling versus standard care, with subsequent in-hospital cooling according to local institutional protocols. Intra-nasal cooling was achieved with a nasal cannula that delivered both a liquid coolant and high-flow oxygen; evaporation of the coolant from the highly vascular nasal mucosa causes the removal of considerable amounts of heat. After an average of 26 min of intra-nasal cooling prior to hospital arrival, tympanic temperature was lowered by 1.3°C and core temperature was nearly 1°C lower in the treatment group versus the controls. Pre-hospital treatment with the intra-nasal cooling system was associated with significantly shorter time to target core temperature (102 min from return of spontaneous circulation in treated subjects versus 289 min in controls) [9]. No statistically significant differences were observed in rates of survival to hospital discharge or neurologic status, but this may be related to study size. This device is not presently available in the United States.

As the body temperature falls, homeostatic mechanisms will tend to generate heat and maintain temperature. Hence, shivering is especially common during induction. Not only does shivering delay induction by generating heat, shivering is associated with marked increases in oxygen requirements and a general hyperadrenergic state, which may exacerbate cardiac irritability [10, 11]. During internal cooling, surface counter-warming with warmed blankets or forced-air blankets (such as the BairHugger, Arizant Healthcare, MN) reduces shivering by raising the temperature of cutaneous cold receptors. Sedatives and analgesics may attenuate shivering. Low doses of meperidine (12.5–25 mg) have been reported to be effective [12] and buspirone, a partial serotonin agonist, has been shown to synergistically reduce shivering in combination with meperidine [13]. Paralysis with pharmaceutical agents such as pancuronium or vecuronium may be required to control shivering and promote rapid induction of therapeutic hypothermia. All of these approaches were employed in the large interventional trials, but comparative data on paralytic agents in the setting of hypothermia post-cardiac arrest and the relative benefits of more rapid induction versus the potential increase in neuromuscular side effects with paralysis have not yet been studied.

During the induction phase, hypercapnea is common, so ventilation should be titrated with frequent arterial blood gas analysis [14]. Other side effects of therapeutic hypothermia, including electrolyte disturbances, hyperglycemia, and seizures, are discussed elsewhere.

Maintenance

Once core hypothermia (32–34°C) is achieved, this temperature should be maintained for 12 h (with ice packs in the Australian study) to 24 h (with cool air in the European study). This requires ongoing cooling in the intensive care unit and precise measurement of core body temperature.

The original trials maintained hypothermia with the same technique used for induction, but as alluded to above, there are situations when separating these stages may be helpful clinically. Infusion of cold saline cannot be continued without causing hypervolemia and immersion methods are efficacious for induction, but can limit access to the patient for procedures, examination, and routine care. Importantly in tertiary care settings, outlying hospitals can start cooling with noninvasive measures and the referral center can maintain hypothermia with techniques that may offer better control of body temperature. The original trials both used external (surface) cooling techniques, but for practical reasons, endovascular techniques may offer specific benefits. A number of commercial devices designed for therapeutic hypothermia are available and briefly described below.

A key consideration in the intensive care unit is access to the patient. Since hypothermia will be maintained for 24 h plus time for rewarming, nurses and physicians will need to examine the patient, place invasive and noninvasive monitoring devices, and possibly perform diagnostic and therapeutic procedures while the temperature management device is in place.

Standard intensive care measures should continue as clinically indicated. Should hypotension or other hemodynamic instability occur, the cause must be sought and treated. Although hypothermia may cause hypotension, rewarming is not generally helpful, as rewarming is associated with vasodilation and may actually worsen hypotension. If hypothermia itself is the cause of hypotension, adequate volume resuscitation and inotropic or vasopressor therapy should be used to support blood pressure.

Re-warming

After a period of 24 h of therapeutic hypothermia, gradual rewarming to normal core temperature (36.5–37.5°C) can begin. When cool air or ice packs are used for maintenance of hypothermia, they can simply be removed and blankets or warm air used to warm the patient. Most commercially available systems automate this process. Applied temperatures (i.e., the temperature of heating blankets) greater than 40°C can cause skin burns and should be avoided. Temperature changes of 0.3–0.5°C/h are generally advocated to allow for equilibration of temperatures throughout the body and avoid over-warming. More rapid changes may provoke marked vasodilation in the periphery, shunting warm blood away from internal organs and paradoxically causing a drop in core temperature a phenomenon referred to as after-drop. Over-shoot rewarming may also be associated with rapid changes in the intracranial pressure and the peripheral vascular resistance, leading to hemodynamic instability and worse neurologic outcomes.

Normothermia should be maintained for the next 24–48 h, as hyperthermia in the post-cardiac arrest period has been correlated with worse neurologic outcomes [15]. In patients with fever, this may simply require antipyretics, but pharmacologic therapies may have limited utility in patients with neurologic injury and continued application of active cooling may be required to maintain normothermia in some patients.

Comparisons Between Techniques

The pivotal clinical trials of therapeutic hypothermia after cardiac arrest used ice packs and an air-circulating cooling blanket; these were not compared to each other directly. A small trial in the Netherlands enrolled 50 consecutive patients with an indication for either therapeutic hypothermia (33 ± 0.2°C) or hyperthermic patients with an indication for strict normothermia (37 ± 0.2°C) and randomized them to five different cooling methods. Cooling with infusion of ice-cold saline and application of ice packs served as the control. Water-circulation cooling system, gel-coated cooling pads, and an intravascular cooling catheter were all associated with more rapid cooling than control but were all similar to each other in terms of rate of cooling; an air-circulating cooling mattress was not substantially different from control, and patients treated with the air-circulating mattress were more likely to require application of additional cooling (ie, with ice packs) to achieve target core temperature. The endovascular system was associated with the least variation in temperature during the study period and with the greatest time in the targeted temperature range, although given the narrow range of target temperature in the study, the significance of this finding is not clear [16]. As the number of patients receiving therapeutic hypothermia and the number of devices available increase, more comparative studies will be important to understand the risks and benefits of different methods.

Commercially-Available Systems

As alluded to above, ad hoc cooling with ice packs or ice cold saline can be effective for therapeutic hypothermia and require no special equipment to implement. However, to achieve a steady temperature of 32–34°C for 24 h, these techniques become cumbersome. Ice cold saline especially is limited in that continuous infusion in the interest of cooling the patient will likely result in volume overload. Ice packs may also pose an infection risk, result in over or under cooling, interfere with patient care in the intensive care unit. To address these limitations, several purpose-made devices have been developed and approved for temperature control in other settings and may be used for therapeutic hypothermia in comatose survivors of cardiac arrest. The available devices fall into two broad categories: external or surface cooling and endovascular cooling. External cooling of blood and returning it to the body, as with cardiopulmonary bypass or the hemodialysis machine, is additionally possible, but not routinely used in survivors of cardiac arrest.

External Systems

External or surface cooling systems generally consist of blankets or pads that are wrapped around the limbs and torso or applied directly to the skin. Systems such as these have been used for temperature control in the operating room for many years. These are noninvasive and therefore carry minimal

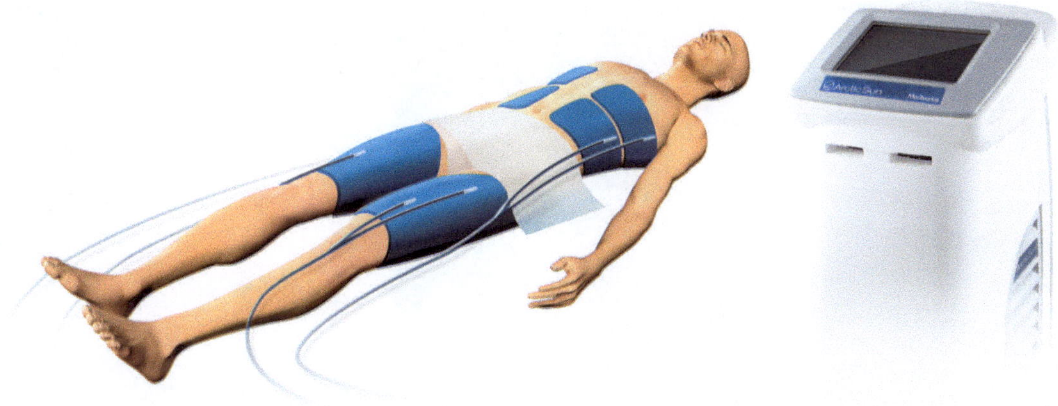

Fig. 5.1 The Arctic Sun gel-pads and temperature management console

bleeding or infection risks. One system, designed specifically for induction of hypothermia, irrigates the skin directly with water.

Arctic Sun (Medivance, Louisville, CO)

The ArcticSun system consists of a console that circulates cooled water through gel-coated pads that are applied to the skin with an adhesive (Fig. 5.1). Single-use, leak-resistant pads are available in several sizes. The direct application to the patient's skin allows the pads to transfer heat by conduction. The pads are radiolucent and safe for MRI environments and therefore do not interfere with diagnostic imaging. The pads should only be applied on intact skin.

Blanketrol (Cincinatti Sub-Zero Products, Cincinnati, OH)

The Blanketrol console can be used with a combination of disposable, water-filled blankets, vests, and headwraps, covering the body with a customized fit (Fig. 5.2). The console circulates cold water through the blankets to control patient temperature noninvasively.

InnerCool STx (Royal Philips Electronics, The Netherlands)

The InnerCool STx circulates cold water through a vest and thigh pads worn by the patient (Fig. 5.3). No adhesive is used. Indwelling esophageal, urinary bladder, and rectal temperature probes are available to allow the console server to titrate cooling to core body temperature.

Medi-Therm (Gaymar Industries, Orchard Park, NY)

The Medi-Therm console circulates water through single-use or reusable conductive water-filled blankets and body wraps that are applied to the patient without an adhesive.

ThermoSuit (LifeRecovery Systems, Kinnelon, NJ)

The ThermoSuit System consists of a body suit that is set up on a patient gurney or bed and the patient placed inside (Fig. 5.4). Cold water is then circulated over and around the patient, in direct contact with the skin. In a multicenter trial, this device was able to cool patients from normothermia (approximately 36°C) to 33°C in an average of 37 min [17]. The system is not designed for maintenance of hypothermia or rewarming but may be ideal for outlying hospitals trying to induce therapeutic hypothermia prior to transfer to a tertiary care center.

Endovascular Systems

Currently available endovascular systems use a catheter with a closed circuit for circulating cold saline through the catheter to cool the blood; no

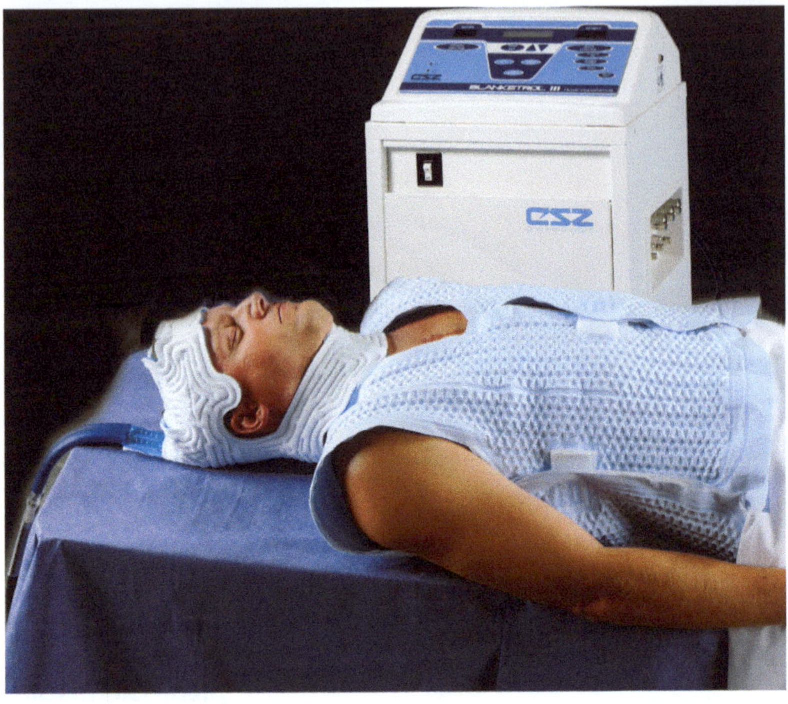

Fig. 5.2 The Blanketrol temperature management system

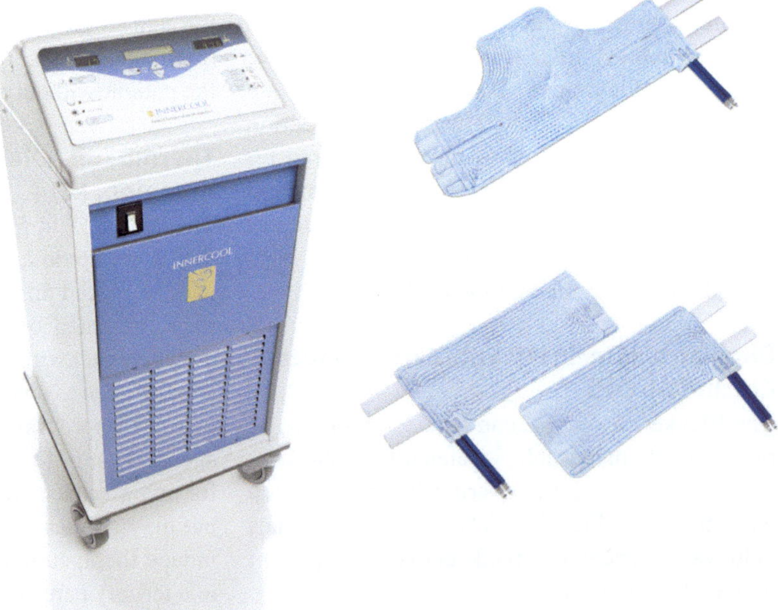

Fig. 5.3 The InnerCool STx cooling blankets and temperature management console

fluid is infused into the patient with these systems. Because insertion of the catheter requires a physician or a midlevel practitioner, these systems are not suitable for use outside of the hospital setting. The placement of a catheter also carries all the usual risks of central venous access, including bleeding, infection, and local trauma, although meticulous critical care can reduce these complications. Endovascular methods may offer increased control of temperature and allow unrestricted access to the patient for routine care and assessment.

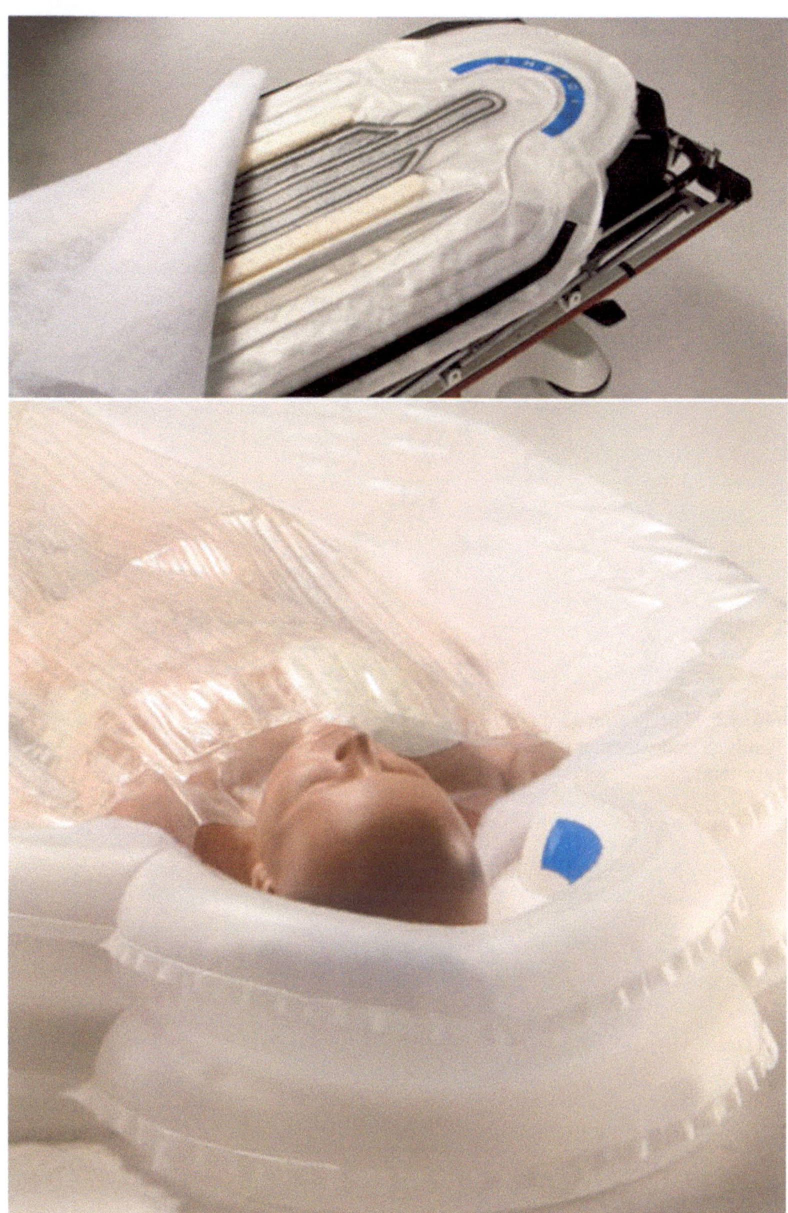

Fig. 5.4 The ThermoSuit immersion cooling device

InnerCool RTx (Formerly Celcius Control; Royal Philips Electronics, The Netherlands)

The InnerCool RTx system uses either a 10.7- or 14-French catheter inserted into a central vein for cooling (Fig. 5.5). The procedure is performed at the bedside using the modified Seldinger technique similar to central venous catheters. The catheter is heparin-coated to prevent thrombosis. Cold saline circulates through the catheter and exchanges heat with the blood stream. Catheters are available with or without temperature probes; if the catheter is used without an integrated temperature probe, the console accepts temperature from a separate temperature probe. The catheter is radio-opaque so that placement can be confirmed radiographically and the manufacturer states that the catheter can safely remain in place for head-only MRIs.

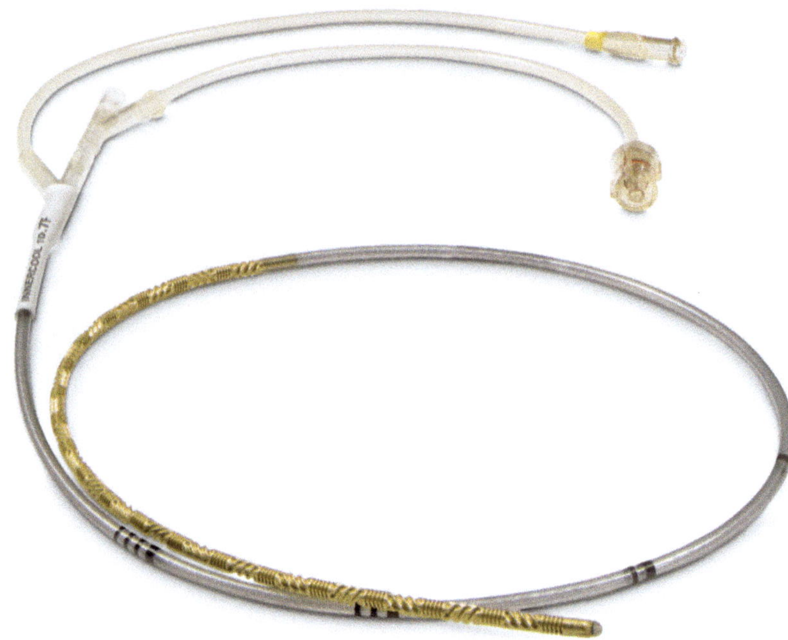

Fig. 5.5 The InnerCool RTx endovascular cooling catheter

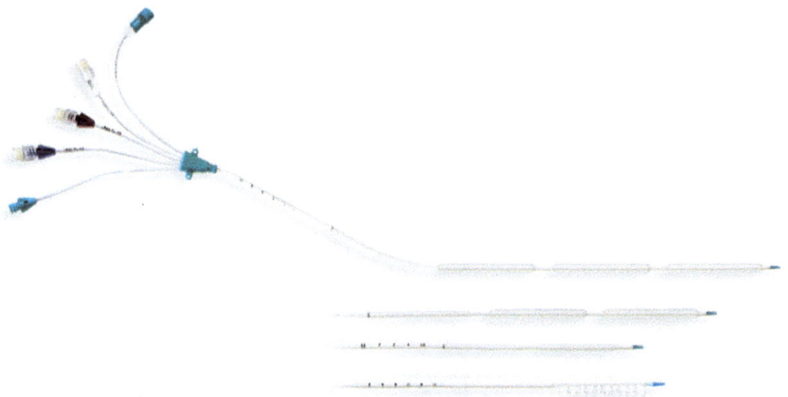

Fig. 5.6 The Thermogard family of endovascular cooling catheters

ThermoGuard (Formerly CoolGard; Zoll Medical Corporation, Chelmsford, MA)

The ThermoGuard system consists of a control console and a range of 9-French catheters with various profiles for central venous insertion (Fig. 5.6). The catheters are heparin-coated to prevent thrombosis. In addition to a closed-loop balloon for heat exchange, the catheters have three lumens for infusion or phlebotomy, similar to a standard central venous catheter. The catheters are radio-opaque and safe for MRI.

Conclusion and Personal Perspective

At our institution, we initiate therapeutic hypothermia with large-volume (30 ml/kg, up to 2 l) infusion of ice-cold (4°C) saline over 30 min. If possible, this is started in the ambulance for comatose patients after out-of-hospital cardiac arrest (see Chap. 2). Patients are then assessed in the emergency department (out-of-hospital cardiac arrests) or in the cardiovascular care unit (in hospital arrests) for contraindications to therapeutic hypothermia (see Chap. 4). Cardiac arrest survivors with evidence of myocardial ischemia are taken emergently to the cardiac catheterization laboratory for coronary angiography and an endovascular temperature control catheter is placed during the procedure. Patients without an emergent indication for cardiac catheterization are taken to the cardiovascular intensive care unit and an endovascular temperature control catheter is placed at the bedside. Temperature is monitored with a probe in the esophagus, rectum or urinary bladder. The goal in all cases is induction of therapeutic hypothermia (core temperature 33°C) as rapidly as possible following the return of spontaneous circulation.

During induction, most patients require meperidine alone or in combination with buspirone or surface counter warming with a forced-air blanket to avoid shivering. If these maneuvers are insufficient to control shivering, we selectively paralyze patients, but we avoid doing so routinely. We routinely administer prophylactic antibiotics to prevent aspiration pneumonia and bloodstream infection. Therapeutic hypothermia is maintained by the endovascular temperature management system for 24 h. The patient is then re-warmed at a rate of 0.5°C every 2 h. Once the patient is normothermic, the endovascular catheter is removed as soon as possible, paralytics and sedatives are stopped, and the patient is extubated as soon as clinically safe. Our center has not observed any increase in catheter-associated blood stream infections despite the use of the intravascular cooling system, possibly owing the use of prophylactic antibiotics.

The presence of the intravascular catheter has only rarely interfered with critical care needs in our institution. Patients without comorbid respiratory diseases can often been weaned from mechanical ventilation quickly if neurologic status is favorable. In cases where neurologic recovery is more protracted, we have a low threshold to involve consultants from neurology. Throughout the hospitalization, involvement of social workers and other support staff are critical for both patients and their families.

References

1. Neumar RW, Nolan JP, Adrie C, Aibiki M, Berg RA, Böttiger BW, et al. Post-cardiac arrest syndrome: epidemiology, pathophysiology, treatment, and prognostication. A consensus statement from the International Liaison Committee on Resuscitation (American Heart Association, Australian and New Zealand Council on Resuscitation, European Resuscitation Council, Heart and Stroke Foundation of Canada, InterAmerican Heart Foundation, Resuscitation Council of Asia, and the Resuscitation Council of Southern Africa); the American Heart Association Emergency Cardiovascular Care Committee; the Council on Cardiovascular Surgery and Anesthesia; the Council on Cardiopulmonary, Perioperative, and Critical Care; the Council on Clinical Cardiology; and the Stroke Council. Circulation. 2008;118:2452–83.
2. Kuboyama K, Safar P, Radovsky A, Tisherman SA, Stezoski SW, Alexander H. Delay in cooling negates the beneficial effect of mild resuscitative cerebral hypothermia after cardiac arrest in dogs: a prospective, randomized study. Crit Care Med. 1993;21(9): 1348–58.
3. Colbourne F, Corbett D. Delayed postischemic hypothermia: a six month survival study using behavioral and histological assessments of neuroprotection. J Neurosci. 1995;15(11):7250–60.
4. Wolff B, Machill K, Schumacher D, Schulzki I, Werner D. Early achievement of mild therapeutic hypothermia and the neurologic outcome after cardiac arrest. Int J Cardiol. 2009;133(2):223–8.
5. Bernard S, Gray T, Buist M, Jones B, Silvester W, Gutteridge G, et al. Treatment of comatose survivors of out-of-hospital cardiac arrest with induced hypothermia. N Engl J Med. 2002;346(8):557–63.
6. The Hypothermia after Cardiac Arrest Study G. Mild therapeutic hypothermia to improve the neurologic outcome after cardiac arrest. N Engl J Med. 2002;346(8): 549–56.
7. Stone JG, Young WL, Smith CR, Solomon RA, Wald A, Ostapkovich N, et al. Do standard monitoring sites reflect true brain temperature when profound hypothermia is rapidly induced and reversed? Anesthesiology. 1995;82(2):344–51.
8. Bernard S, Buist M, Monteiro O, Smith K. Induced hypothermia using large volume, ice-cold intravenous fluid in comatose survivors of out-of-hospital cardiac arrest: a preliminary report. Resuscitation. 2003;56(1):9–13.
9. Castrén M, Nordberg P, Svensson L, Taccone F, Vincent J-L, Desruelles D, et al. Intra-arrest transnasal evaporative cooling: a randomized, prehospital, multicenter study (PRINCE: Pre-ROSC IntraNasal Cooling Effectiveness). Circulation. 2010;122(7):729–36.
10. Frank SM, Fleisher LA, Olson KF, Gorman RB, Higgins MS, Breslow MJ, et al. Multivariate determinants of early postoperative oxygen consumption in elderly patients. Effects of shivering, body temperature, and gender. Anesthesiology. 1995;83(2):241–9.

11. Frank SM, Fleisher LA, Breslow MJ, Higgins MS, Olson KF, Kelly S, et al. Perioperative maintenance of normothermia reduces the incidence of morbid cardiac events. A randomized clinical trial. JAMA. 1997;277(14):1127–34.
12. Polderman KH. Application of therapeutic hypothermia in the intensive care unit. Opportunities and pitfalls of a promising treatment modality–part 2: practical aspects and side effects. Intensive Care Med. 2004;30(5):757–69.
13. Mokhtarani M, Mahgoub AN, Morioka N, Doufas AG, Dae M, Shaughnessy TE. Buspirone and meperidine synergistically reduce the shivering threshold. Anesth Analg. 2001;93(5):1233–9.
14. Falkenbach P, Kämäräinen A, Mäkelä A, Kurola J, Varpula T, Ala-Kokko T, et al. Incidence of iatrogenic dyscarbia during mild therapeutic hypothermia after successful resuscitation from out-of-hospital cardiac arrest. Resuscitation. 2009;80(9):990–3.
15. Zeiner A, Holzer M, Sterz F, Schörkhuber W, Eisenburger P, Havel C, et al. Hyperthermia after cardiac arrest is associated with an unfavorable neurologic outcome. Arch Intern Med. 2001;161(16):2007–12.
16. Hoedemaekers CW, Ezzahti M, Gerritsen A, van der Hoeven JG. Comparison of cooling methods to induce and maintain normo- and hypothermia in intensive care unit patients: a prospective intervention study. Crit Care. 2007;11(4):R91.
17. Howes D, Ohley W, Dorian P, Klock C, Freedman R, Schock R, et al. Rapid induction of therapeutic hypothermia using convective-immersion surface cooling: safety, efficacy and outcomes. Resuscitation. 2010;81(4):388–92.

6 How to Implement Therapeutic Hypothermia in the Hospital

Lisa Hawksworth

Bringing a therapeutic hypothermia program into a hospital involves clinical knowledge, the capital and supply chain process, and the ability to demonstrate a return on investment. As clinicians, we know how to review the literature and incorporate best practice recommendations. Many smaller hospitals have sent patients to larger regional centers to receive therapeutic hypothermia. The benefits to patients are clear and pre-hospital personnel may already know the protocol. Considering a change to keep your patients in your facility rather than shipping them out for hypothermia? The regional centers have seen benefit in downstream revenue that has made this a profitable service to provide. Let's review how to look at your facility and see if bringing a hypothermia program in-house could be worthwhile.

Literature Review

Little is in the published literature about implementing a therapeutic hypothermia program. One useful article from Bruce Jancin described an initiative to create level 1 cardiac arrest centers that "coordinate emergent percutaneous coronary intervention, rapid hypothermia of patients who are comatose or unable to respond appropriately at arrival to the hospital, optimal management in an ICU, and electrophysiologic evaluation with placement of an implanted cardioverter-defibrillator if warranted, and aggressive risk-reduction measures" [1]. This model was presented by Dr. Keith Lurie at the annual scientific sessions of the American Heart Association. Dr. Lurie was able to determine a cost-effectiveness analysis to show a direct average net margin of approximately $20K per survivor and $3K per non-survivor.

In 2009, The Joint Commission convened a stakeholder meeting of key leaders from various organizations, and priority areas related to sudden cardiac arrest were suggested utilizing a multi-focused approach. In February 2010, the Technical Advisory Panel was convened to further refine these priority areas. Preliminary priority areas targeted for measure identification include:

- Use of therapeutic hypothermia
  - Proportion of out of hospital cardiac arrest patients treated with hypothermia in the hospital
  - Time to initiation of cooling
  - If no capability, fast transfer
  - Overuse, underuse, or appropriate use of therapeutic hypothermia [2]

Under the Patient Protection and Affordable Care Act of 2010, Title III is the Value Based Purchasing Program (VBP). It is reasonable to expect that comparative outcomes for patients suffering in-house cardiac arrests may become part of the VBP process-of-care measures and affect the scoring methodology for hospitals that receive Medicare funding.

Another excellent article by Dr. Raina Merchant et al. calculated cost-effectiveness of

L. Hawksworth, MSN, RN, NE-BC
Cardiovascular Services, Mary Washington Healthcare, Fredericksburg, VA, USA
e-mail: lisa.hawksworth@mwhc.com

J.B. Lundbye (ed.), *Therapeutic Hypothermia After Cardiac Arrest*, DOI 10.1007/978-1-4471-2951-6_6, © Springer-Verlag London 2012 postresuscitation costs accrued by survivors of cardiac arrest based on quality adjusted life years (QALY). They concluded that:

> Even if a hospital had only 1 patient eligible for hypothermia annually, and considerable postresuscitation care costs were accrued by survivors the cost-effectiveness of hypothermia would remain less than $100,000/ QALY. This level of cost-effectiveness is consistent with many widely accepted health care interventions and is considerably lower than some other estimates of US societal willingness to pay for health care [3].

Since most hospitals do not evaluate cost-effectiveness of programs based on QALY but rather based on direct return on investment to the facility, a cost-benefit analysis will need to be performed prior to implementation of a therapeutic hypothermia program.

Know Your Numbers

If your hospital is regularly bypassed by Emergency Medical Services (EMS) personnel, you may not be able to accurately measure the full impact of a therapeutic hypothermia program until after implementation. “Feeder hospitals” provide volume sources for regional cooling centers. These centers have successfully promoted their services and positive outcomes to outlying hospitals. Working with EMS to modify bypass protocols after implementation of a therapeutic hypothermia program will be critical in measuring return on investment for your facility.

Knowing your in-house cardiac arrest volume and outcomes will provide a starting point for calculating the effect a cooling program can provide. The National Registry of CardioPulmonary Resuscitation (NRCPR) provides a national benchmark for in-house cardiac arrest outcomes. In 2009, the U.S. national average for intact neurologic survival post-cardiac arrest was 20%.

Numbers to know:

1. Number of codes per year
2. Number of codes that survive to ICU
3. Number of patients that survive to 24 h
4. Number of patients that survive to discharge
5. Number that survive from ICU neurologically intact
6. Number of patients with care withdrawn/or Do Not Resuscitate (DNR) from ICU

Consider how your in-house arrest data compares to national average. Consider how well your hospital manages patients based on their neurologic outcomes. Do your patients have better than average neurologic outcomes post-cardiac arrest? Being able to define your pre-implementation outcomes will help you quantify the impact on your patients and the impact on your community.

Benefits

The goal of a therapeutic hypothermia program is to optimize the neurologic outcome of patients suffering out-of-house and in-house cardiac arrest. Successful adoption of a therapeutic hypothermia program will help retain cardiac patient volume that may have been bypassing your facility thereby generating new cardiac patient volume. In addition, in-house cardiac arrest patients will have a higher likelihood of neurologic recovery and generate increased revenue from additional cardiac procedures such as CABG, PTCA and ICD placement (Fig. 6.1).

Calculating Market Demand

As a hospital not offering therapeutic hypothermia, unless you have bypass data from your EMS providers, market demand for therapeutic hypothermia for out-of-house cardiac arrest must be calculated through indirect means. Your hospital may not currently receive all of the out-of-house cardiac arrest patient population from your EMS providers if they have a bypass protocol for therapeutic hypothermia.

Since cardiac disease is the primary cause of cardiac arrest in adults, market forecasts for the change in patient services requiring cardiac care can give a level of indication as to the need for therapeutic hypothermia for out-of-house cardiac arrest. Population projections can be forecast and coupled with the aging of the population and the increased likelihood of cardiac arrest with aging, your hospital’s market demand for therapeutic hypothermia in the post-cardiac arrest patient can be estimated.

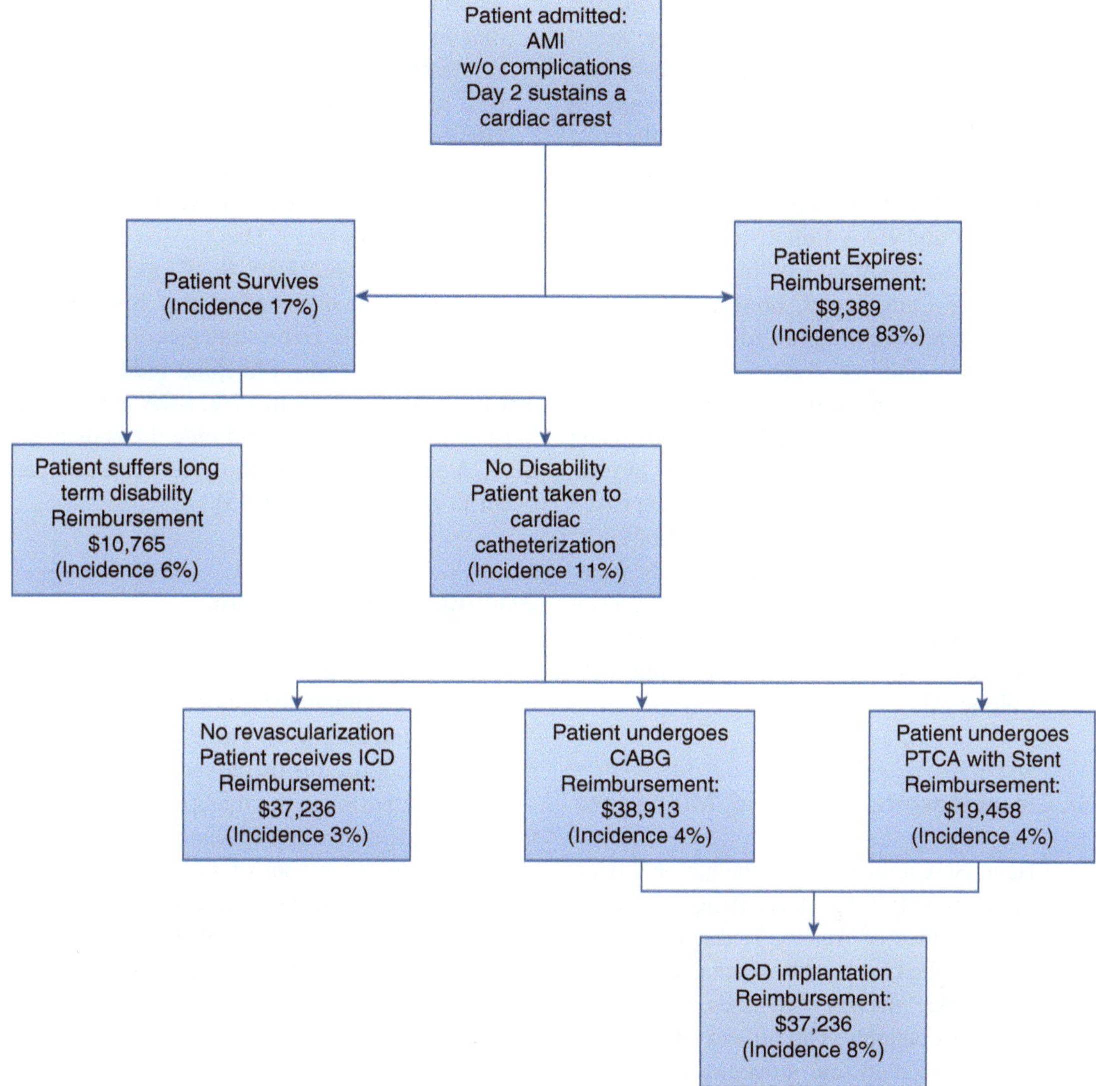

Fig. 6.1 Financial analysis tool (Modified from Ref. [1])

Know Your Competition

How competitive is your healthcare marketplace? Do you have several local competitors already receiving patients for cooling from EMS? How far would a cardiac arrest patient in the field have to travel to be cooled? Is positioning your hospital as a Center for Cardiac Excellence and a referral center for complex cardiac care in your strategic planning for your facility? Demonstrated superior patient neurologic outcomes from a "level one cardiac arrest center" would be highly marketable in a multi-hospital community.

Benchmarks

VCU Medical Center and Richmond Ambulance Authority

Virginia Commonwealth University (VCU) Medical Center and the Richmond Ambulance

Authority (RAA) have improved resuscitation and survival rates dramatically for cardiac arrest patients by training and equipping paramedics to begin lowering a patient's body temperature in the field during resuscitation and following up at the hospital with a host of high-tech strategies to improve the odds of survival [4].

The VCU and RAA initiative, known as the Advanced Resuscitation Cooling Therapeutics and Intensive Care Center, or ARCTIC, is the most comprehensive program of its kind in the United States, and its strategy resulted in an almost twofold improvement in the return of spontaneous circulation, from 25% in 2001 using conventional treatments to 46% in 2008. In turn, the survival rate to hospital discharge improved from 9.7% in 2003 to 17.9% at the end of 2008. The national average is less than 7%. The comprehensive ARCTIC approach is showing greater benefit than that which was seen using just conventional resuscitation and simple cooling techniques alone [4].

St. Cloud Hospital, St. Cloud, Minnesota

Take Heart St. Cloud is part of the national demonstration project, Take Heart America, which includes the cities of Austin, Texas; Columbus, Ohio; and Anoka County, Minnesota. Take Heart celebrates twice the survival rates for Sudden Cardiac Arrest patients. The project has simultaneously implemented four strategies to improve out-of-hospital sudden cardiac arrest survival rates. Strategies include:

- Teaching cardiopulmonary resuscitation/automated external defibrillator (CPR/AED) education and training to all high school freshmen and to the community at-large in a wide-spread education effort to increase CPR/AED skills;
- Deployment of AEDs in strategically positioned locations to maximize bystander access;
- Comprehensive professional rescuer training (emergency medical practitioners and emergency/trauma room personnel) with newly recommended CPR techniques and devices that double circulation during CPR;
- Implementation of specific treatments for post-resuscitation care after successful resuscitation, including systemic hypothermia for unconscious survivors, and aggressive evaluation and treatment with interventional cardiology techniques and ICDs.

Data from Take Heart St. Cloud and Take Heart Anoka County confirm that implementation of the four Take Heart strategies does increase survivability from out-of-hospital sudden cardiac arrest (SCA) from 9% to 17%. SCA is the number one killer of women and men. Less than 5% of SCA victims leave the hospital alive and can occur in people of all ages [5].

Pricing/Reimbursement

Patients using temperature management modalities will be reimbursed under the traditional DRGs for their diagnosis. There is not additional reimbursement for this therapy at this time.

The incentive to use this therapy is derived from the increased positive clinical neurologic outcomes and the future alignment of favorable outcomes with increased reimbursement (Fig. 6.2).

There is an increase in reimbursement that has been noted by centers that have implemented all the strongest recommendations of the 2005 AHA resuscitation guidelines. The key elements of care provided at "level one cardiac arrest centers" are emergent percutaneous coronary intervention, rapid hypothermia of patients who are comatose or unable to respond appropriately upon arrival at the hospital, optimal management in the ICU, electrophysiologic evaluation along with placement of an implantable cardiac defibrillator if warranted, and aggressive risk-reduction measures [6]. These centers have shown dramatic increase in discharge rates of patients suffering out of hospital cardiac arrest, well above the national average. In addition, they have been able to quantify an increase in reimbursement for survivors of in-house spontaneous cardiac arrest (SCA). St. Cloud Hospital in Minnesota was able to demonstrate an average revenue increase of $48,483

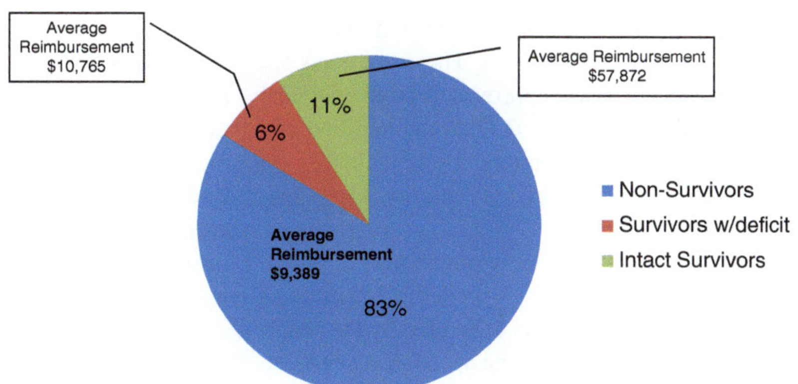

Fig. 6.2 Net reimbursement (Modified from Ref. [1])

per patient of neurologically intact survivors who went on to receive additional procedures (CABG, PTCA with stent, ICD implant) [5].

Based on this formula, your hospital can calculate the average difference in reimbursement that would be gained for incremental survivors with positive neurologic outcome as a result of therapeutic hypothermia post-cardiac arrest (Fig. 6.2).

A study by Merchant et al., demonstrated that the incremental cost-effectiveness ratio of therapeutic hypothermia was $47,168 per quality-adjusted life year compared with conventional care [3]. They concluded that hypothermia in cardiac arrest patients improved clinical outcomes with cost-effectiveness comparable to many economically acceptable health care interventions in the United States.

Operational Structure

Consider how therapeutic hypothermia will be implemented in your facility. Perhaps the proposed clinical modifications will require a patient admitted post out-of-hospital cardiac arrest to be sent to the Cardiac Catheterization Lab for care to include insertion of a hypothermia catheter and early initiation of therapeutic hypothermia. If the patient is an in-house cardiac arrest, the patient will be brought to the ICU for post-code care and initiation of therapeutic hypothermia via the hypothermia catheter or via external cooling devices.

Therapeutic hypothermia will be maintained for 24 h and then the patient will be rewarmed according to protocol and either maintained on normothermia protocol or allowed to self-thermoregulate. The temperature management system should only be used in the ICU. Patients requiring therapeutic hypothermia must be intubated and sedated during the hypothermic phase of care. Patients requiring maintenance of normothermia via the intravascular cooling device may be considered for extubation as tolerated as the device does not create patient shivering as external cooling devices do. Patients that shiver rewarm themselves and counteract the temperature maintenance function of the catheters, usually requiring sedation or other medication to counteract the shivering.

Process changes may include the following:

- Flowchart: timeline to guide therapy
- Therapeutic Hypothermia Order Set: to be used for all patients needing therapeutic hypothermia
- Guidelines for Induced Hypothermia for Resuscitated Victims of Cardiac Arrest: evidence-based clinical references for bedside providers
- Policies: to document standards

Capital Equipment

The capital equipment required for therapeutic hypothermia will include cooling consoles. The remaining equipment will be disposables and other non-capital supplies. There are usually options other than outright purchase of the capital equipment to facilitate implementation of a therapeutic hypothermia program. These contracts are typically reviewed and approved through a Clinical Quality Value Analysis (CQVA) committee and the hospital legal department. These include:

1. **Disposable upcharge agreements**. These usually require a purchase order to guarantee a preset number of disposable purchases per month over a defined period. A predefined number of consoles would be able to be used by the hospital during the period of the upcharge agreement. At the end of the defined period or purchase of the full number of disposables at the upcharge rate, whichever comes first, the consoles would be paid for and belong to the hospital. Ideally, the upcharge agreement could have a no-fault cancellation clause where the hospital could notify the vendor of the intent to stop the program, finish using all remaining shipped disposables and arrange for return of the consoles to the vendor, but these are not typical.

   Using disposable cost, minimum additional cost per patient under the upcharge agreement can be determined.
2. **Console purchase**. More typical are traditional console purchase agreements where the consoles are purchased and delivered for immediate use. The consoles may be financed over time with the vendor. Disposables will also need to be purchased for the equipment and may be included in the console purchase agreement or separately.
3. **Fleet conversion discount.** Depending on the vendor, there may be potential to include therapeutic hypothermia consoles as a part of a fleet conversion for multiple types of equipment made by that vendor. For example, since Zoll makes both temperature management consoles and defibrillators, there may be opportunity to negotiate additional discounts with larger purchase agreements to include multiple items in a vendor's fleet. The price of the console may be absorbed such a proposal.

Staffing

Due to the decreased workload on nursing, patients with temperature management devices can be managed at current ICU nurse-to-patient ratios based on other critical patient characteristics (vasoactive medications, etc.). Temperature management devices have been shown to decrease nursing workload associated with fever management in ICU settings due to their active modulation of temperature in response to the patient's core temperature [7]. As the hospital looks to improve efficiency in ICU staffing, temperature management devices can assist in that effort.

Education

The clinical expertise and competency of the nurses in the ICU to care for the patient with a therapeutic hypothermia device is essential to the success of the program. The vendor will usually provide education from clinical specialists during the go-live period of the agreement. The training will need to be integrated into annual skills training until this is no longer a low-volume procedure. Cardiac Cath Lab nurses may also need to be included in the training if they begin the hypothermia process in the Cath Lab. Training cost can be calculated with the average hourly wage of the nurses and the number of nurses to train with estimates from the clinical team on initial and ongoing training hours. Usually a core team is trained during the initial implementation of the program and then as the therapy becomes more widely used, the rest of the nursing staff are trained. The vendor should include ongoing support and education.

Physicians in the Cath Lab and ICU will need to be trained on the device as well. If the intravascular therapeutic hypothermia device is selected, the physicians will need to be trained to insert the device as well as their midlevel practitioners. This training should also be included in the educational go-live from the vendor. Insertion of the intravascular device is similar to other central line insertions and is not complex for the physicians to learn.

Return on Investment

In order for therapeutic hypothermia program to break even on the hospital investment the number needed to treat will need to be calculated. If

Codes per year	Incremental Survival	Incremental $ per year
20	4	$193,932
50	7	$339,381
200	40	$1,939,320
300	60	$2,908,980

Fig. 6.3 Cash flow impact of improving outcomes. The number is obtained by subtracting reimbursement (non-survivor) from reimbursement (survivor). This is then multiplied by the increase in number of intact survivors (Modified from Ref [1])

one of these patients improved their neurologic outcome, the revenue gained would be calculated as the difference in reimbursement between intact survivors and non-survivors (Fig. 6.3).

Knowing your baseline success with neurologic outcomes post cardiac arrest will help determine your likely improvement in neurologic outcomes through implementing a therapeutic hypothermia program. If you have already had some success in neurologic outcomes through standard resuscitation, the likelihood of improved actual return on investment will be much greater. In addition, the decrease in the out-migration of cardiac arrest patients will improve the bottom line in your cardiac service line.

Critical Success Factors

In order to achieve the benefits/outcomes previously identified, the program must have intensive collaboration of the multidisciplinary team of professionals, including EMS providers; ED nurses, physicians and staff; Cath Lab nurses, physicians and staff; the Rapid Response Team; ICU nurses, physicians and staff, Biomedical Engineering and Supply Chain Management.

Impact on Hospital Mission and Vision

Providing the cardiac and intensive care that produces the best neurologic outcomes for patients will distinguish your facility as a regional leader in cardiac care. Review your hospital's mission and vision statement to see if implementing therapeutic hypothermia would assist in fulfilling the mission and vision. The therapeutic hypothermia program will:

- Increase the survival of out-of-hospital cardiac arrest patients
- Improve the neurologic outcomes of in-house cardiac arrest patients to that of top performing hospitals

References

1. Jancin B. Cardiac arrest centers boost survival, profits. www.ecardiologynews.com. 2009; 7:1, 9.
2. The Joint Commission. Performance measurement initiatives sudden cardiac arrest call for performance measures. (2010). http://www.jointcommission.org/PerformanceMeasurement/PerformanceMeasurement/Sudden+Cardiac+Arrest+–+Call+for+Perf+Meas.htm. Accessed 17 Mar 2010.
3. Merchant RM, Becker LB, Abella BS, Asch DA, Groeneveld PW. Cost-effectiveness of therapeutic hypothermia after cardiac arrest. Circ Cardiovasc Qual Outcomes. 2009;2:421–8.
4. Virginia Commonwealth University Medical Center. Resuscitation and survival rates from out-of-hospital cardiac arrest nearly double with comprehensive treatment protocol (2009). http://www.news.vcu.edu/news/Resuscitation_and_Survival_Rates_from_OutofHospital_Cardiac_Arrest. Accessed 16 Nov 2009.
5. CentraCare Health System. Take Heart celebrates twice the survival rates for Sudden Cardiac Arrest patients (2008).http://www.centracare.com/community/media_releases/take_heart_stcloud_celebrates_survival_rates.html. Accessed 21 Oct 2008.
6. Hypothermia after Cardiac Arrest Study Group. Mild therapeutic hypothermia to improve the neurologic

outcome after cardiac arrest. N Engl J Med. 2002;346(8):549–56.

7. Lemons N. University of Alabama at Birmingham comprehensive Stroke Center. Novel intravascular heat exchange central venous catheter reduces fever and nursing time associated with neuro intensive care patients. Abstract presentation for AACN Region 6 Meeting. 27 Sept 2004.

7 Post-cardiac Arrest: How to Develop and Implement a Standard Therapeutic Hypothermia Protocol?

Sanjeev U. Nair, Xia Luo, and Justin B. Lundbye

Introduction

Therapeutic Hypothermia (TH) for post-cardiac arrest management is becoming standard therapy since it has been shown to improve neurologic and survival outcomes in cardiac arrest survivors. Two ground-breaking prospective trials in 2002 showed that inducing hypothermia in patients who were successfully resuscitated from cardiac arrest due to ventricular fibrillation (VF) resulted in better neurologic recovery and survival of these patients [1, 2]. Following these and subsequent studies which showed promising results with TH in cardiac arrest survivors, the International Liaison Committee on Resuscitation (ILCOR) and the American Heart Association (AHA) issued guidelines that recommend the use of mild therapeutic hypothermia (32–34°C) for 12–24 h in all cardiac arrest survivors [3, 4].

The principle of cooling cardiac arrest survivors is simple, but its implementation in the field as well as the hospital setting remains challenging. Establishing a standard protocol and order set to manage all necessary elements of this therapy is the best way to ensure successful utilization of TH for institutions. A team approach is essential for the successful development and implementation of a TH protocol. Key elements when developing a successful TH protocol include:

- Identifying physician and nursing champions on the TH team
- Support and collaboration within multiple departments (Emergency Medicine, Critical Care, Cardiology, Neurology, Pulmonary)
- Establishing interdisciplinary support from Pharmacy, Biomedical engineering, Respiratory therapy, Infection Control, and Laboratory Medicine
- Establishing regular work meetings for the protocol development team to discuss the available literature on the subject, funding resources, equipment availability, and method of cooling, education of personnel, as well as impediments in each stage of protocol implementation.

This chapter serves as a guide to provide key steps in the development and implementation of a TH protocol in a hospital setting.

Guidelines in Developing the TH Protocol

The primary task of the TH protocol development team involves establishing crucial steps to ensure successful implementation. The TH protocol team

S.U. Nair, MBBS, M.D., FACP (✉)
J.B. Lundbye, M.D., FACC
Division of Cardiology, Henry Low Heart Center, Hartford Hospital, Hartford, CT, USA
e-mail: sunair@harthosp.org

University of Connecticut School of Medicine, Farmington, CT, USA
e-mail: jlundbye@thocc.org

X. Luo, M.D.
Clinical Education, ZOLL, Sunnyvale, CA, USA
e-mail: xluo@zoll.com

J.B. Lundbye (ed.), *Therapeutic Hypothermia After Cardiac Arrest*,
DOI 10.1007/978-1-4471-2951-6_7, © Springer-Verlag London 2012

will need to first develop inclusion and exclusion criteria for patient selection. Second, they will need to determine where the TH therapy will be initiated (Emergency Department, Intensive Care Unit or by Emergency Medical Services). Third, the team will need to discuss various methods of cooling. Finally, the team will need to establish guidelines on routine patient monitoring and possible side effects related to the TH procedure.

Patient Selection

The AHA has updated guidelines on post-cardiac arrest care in 2010. Recommendations include [3]:

1. Comatose (i.e. lack of meaningful response to verbal commands) adult patients with return of spontaneous circulation (ROSC) after out-of-hospital VF cardiac arrest should be cooled to 32–34°C (89.6–93.2°F) for 12–24 h (Class I, LOE B).
2. Induced hypothermia may also be considered for comatose adult patients with ROSC after in-hospital cardiac arrest of any initial rhythm or after out-of-hospital cardiac arrest with an initial rhythm of pulseless electric activity or asystole (Class IIb, LOE B).

Based on these guidelines, all cardiac arrest survivors should be considered for TH therapy. However, the protocol must include both relative and absolute exclusions based on consensus. For example, patients with a do-not-resuscitate order, advanced malignancy, and those who are pregnant are typically excluded from TH therapy by most institutions.

Initiation of TH

The protocol should state where the cooling of a patient is to be initiated. Most emergency medical services are now able to cool cardiac arrest patients using ice cold saline and ice packs en route to the hospital. If the determination has been made by the TH protocol team to cool the patient by internal methods, the protocol needs to state clearly who is responsible for placing the cooling catheter to begin therapy (Emergency physician, Intensivist, Interventionalist). Moreover, if the patient needs urgent cardiac catheterization, the protocol should state whether internal cooling should be initiated prior to or after cardiac catheterization.

Method of Cooling

External and internal cooling methods have been shown to be feasible and effective in lowering core body temperature to the target range of 32–34°C (89.6–93.2°F) [5–7]. The system that is utilized must have a continuous temperature monitoring and feedback mechanism in order to prevent inadequate or excessive cooling. External cooling devices include cooling pads or mattresses. Some surface pads are easy to apply and can be initiated by the nursing staff. This method involves covering as much body surface area as possible. During external cooling, the skin condition should be closely monitored for signs of frostnip and managed appropriately. Intravascular cooling devices include a central line insertion, either by subclavian, internal jugular, or femoral line placement. The decision regarding the method of cooling involves financial and practical aspects of implementation. Endovascular cooling may be more expensive due to the cost of disposable catheters. On the other hand although costs may be cut down by using only external cooling, this form of cooling may be less efficient in achieving target temperatures as compared to endovascular cooling [6]. The TH team should base the selection of method of cooling by considering all phases of the TH procedure: time to reach and maintain tight control of the target temperature, ability to control the rewarming phase, and prevention of rebound hyperthermia in the post-rewarming (normothermia) phase.

Selection of Target Temperature, Length of TH Procedure and Rewarming

The ILCOR and AHA recommend that patients be cooled to a target temperature range of 32–34°C for 12–24 h. Bernard et al. [2] cooled patients to 33°C for 12 h and in the HACA trial [1] patients were cooled to 32–34°C for 24 h. Both studies demonstrated survival and neurologic benefits. However, the absolute optimal target temperature and duration of cooling are yet to be determined.

The rewarming phase should be slow and controlled. The AHA most recently has recommended that rewarming be done at a rate of 0.25°C/h. Rebound hyperthermia should be avoided once normothermia has been achieved.

Core Body Temperature Monitoring

It is vital to have a robust mechanism in order to continuously monitor the core body temperature while cooling, as well as while rewarming the patient. The placement of thermistors in the esophagus or urinary bladder has been shown to accurately reflect the core body temperature [8]. The use of pulmonary catheter thermistors to monitor core body temperature, although considered the gold standard, is mostly impractical unless they are already in place for hemodynamic monitoring. Peripheral monitoring of temperature i.e. external ear, axilla, or oral is unreliable and not recommended. Thus the TH protocol should include only those forms of temperature monitoring that have been shown to be consistent and accurate.

Hemodynamic Monitoring

Use of central venous line and arterial catheter placement should be considered in cardiac arrest patients undergoing TH in order to help with hemodynamic monitoring. This is especially important due to variations in blood pressure which commonly occur during the induction and maintenance phases of cooling. Moreover there is usually a need for vasopressor/ inotropic support in order to maintain adequate cardiac output during the various phases of TH therapy. Typically, there is also a need for frequent arterial blood gas measurements since cardiac arrest patients usually have acidemia on presentation. The placement of arterial catheters should be done prior to or during the induction phase of cooling since cold-induced vasoconstriction makes this difficult in the later stages of TH.

Ventilatory Management

Use of standard ventilator bundle and prophylactic antibiotics should be implemented in order to prevent ventilator associated pneumonia (VAP) [9, 10]. Since some ventilators have temperature control, the setting should be adjusted to avoid being counterproductive to the cooling and warming phase. Continuous pulse oximetry is required in patients who are undergoing TH. Forehead oximeters have been shown to be reliable in cooled patients and are recommended since peripheral vasoconstriction leads to inaccurate finger oximetry measurements [11].

Neurologic Monitoring

Frequent neurologic monitoring for seizure is advocated since these patients are prone to ischemic seizures which may be masked by the use of paralytics to prevent shivering. Continuous EEG monitoring would be ideal but is not popular due to lack of nurses/technicians trained to interpret continuous EEG tracings.

Infection Control

Patients undergoing TH are at risk of infection secondary to a cooling-induced immunocompromised state. Strict adherence to sterile techniques during catheterization, prompt removal of catheters once their use is over, as well as taking steps to prevent VAP are important in preventing infectious complications.

Staff Education and Implementation of the TH Protocol

Staff education must include the benefits, the potential side effects, the physiological changes and complications of TH. A thorough education plan for the nursing staff involved in running the TH protocol and order set in the intensive care unit is necessary. The key areas for specialized education of nursing and technical staff during the implementation of TH are briefly discussed below.

Hemodynamics and Electrocardiography

Patients undergoing cooling usually have a lowering of the heart rate and changes in blood pressure. Inotropic support for low blood pressure measurements may be required, although most patients require only minimal support to maintain an adequate mean arterial pressure. Prolongation of PR, QRS and QT intervals are also seen in these patients, but they are rarely the primary cause for arrhythmias.

Electrolytes and Acid–Base Balance

Cooling causes the intracellular shift of potassium and a replacement protocol should be implemented in order to avoid arrhythmias. However, during the rewarming phase, caution must be exercised with replacement of potassium since the sequestered potassium moves back into the circulation and can cause toxicity. Low temperatures reduce the release as well as efficacy of anti-diuretic hormone (ADH) and thus a "cold diuresis" occurs that may cause volume and electrolyte depletion. Thus, magnesium, calcium and phosphate levels also need frequent monitoring during the TH therapy. Initial metabolic acidosis in cardiac arrest patients usually corrects over time with the establishment of circulation as long as there is adequate perfusion and ventilation. Due to a predominant fat catabolism during hypothermia, there may be a mild metabolic acidosis due to free fatty acids in the circulation. Cooling causes a reduction of carbon dioxide production and thus aggressive correction of initial respiratory acidosis can lead to alkalosis.

Hyperglycemia

Hypothermia leads to insulin resistance and so higher doses of insulin may be required. Modification of the insulin sliding scale may be necessary in order to control hyperglycemia in patients undergoing TH therapy. Alternatively, during the rewarming phase, the insulin dose will need reduction in order to avoid hypoglycemia. Blood sugars should be monitored using arterial or venous blood since capillary blood sugar estimation is unreliable as a result of peripheral vasoconstriction.

Shivering

Shivering is a physiologic phenomenon and is a common occurrence in cardiac arrest patients undergoing TH. Since it produces heat, increases oxygen consumption, and increases metabolic demands, there may be attenuation or negation of the benefits of cooling. Shivering can be reduced or stopped by the use of sedatives, cutaneous counter- warming and paralytic agents. Institutions differ in the use of these anti-shivering methods in their TH protocol and may either utilize them prophylactically or only with the occurrence of shivering. Paralytics may mask seizure activity and thus patients will need continuous EEG monitoring if these agents are used frequently.

Avoiding Rebound Hyperthermia

Rewarming after the cooling phase should be done slowly and requires close monitoring in order to avoid rebound hyperthermia. Rebound hyperthermia has been associated with poor neurologic outcomes [12]. The use of continuous feedback systems can assist in rewarming patients and maintaining normothermia after the rewarming phase is over. Regular monitoring of electrolytes, blood sugars, as well as hemodynamics is also required during and after the rewarming phase in order to avoid complications like hyperkalemia, hypoglycemia and hypotension respectively.

Post-implementation Monitoring

After implementation of the TH protocol, continuous surveillance of its efficacy as well as regular updates from staff running the protocol is required. A committee for the oversight of the TH therapy should be in place with regularly scheduled meetings. This committee should also include key personnel from other committees which review cardiac arrests and rapid responses in the hospital. To keep the protocol up to date with the available evidence, a constant scrutiny of newly published literature should be performed. Sharing and learning from each other's successes and experiences, which may also include interacting with other institutions in the area should be encouraged.

Conclusions

The use of TH in cardiac arrest survivors is now recommended by the AHA as a standard of care. The development and implementation of a TH protocol in order to achieve maximum therapeutic efficacy utilizing the least amount of resources is challenging. A systematic and collaborative approach using multidisciplinary personnel is the key to designing and carrying out the TH protocol. Regular meetings and rigorous staff education during the initial stage of setting up the protocol will assist in the smooth introduction of TH into practice. Post-implementation surveillance is required to maintain the efficiency and cost-effectiveness of the TH protocol.

The Appendix shows a sample TH protocol/order set based on practice followed at Hartford Hospital. Several other institutions have provided samples of TH protocol on their websites. You can visit:
www.med.upenn.edu/resuscitation/hypothermia/protocols
www.wakeems.com/saem

Appendix

Hartford Hospital Therapeutic Hypothermia Protocol/Order Set

Inclusion/Exclusion criteria must be completed prior to initiating therapy

- Inclusion criteria:
  - Survivors of cardiac arrest (inpatient or outpatient)
  - Unresponsive (defined as total Glasgow coma scale (GCS) <8 or motor score <4 if intubated)
  - Blood pressure >90 mm of Hg systolic (with our without vasopressors)
  - Intubated
- Exclusion criteria:
  - Patients who are do-not-resuscitate (DNR) status
  - Significant immunologic compromise (e.g. AIDS, Leukemia)
  - Active sepsis
  - Hemodynamic instability
  - Down time >30 min to first responder (a relative contraindication)
  - Active bleeding (a relative contraindication)
  - Causes of coma other than cardiac arrest/hypoxic encephalopathy

1. Initiate Patient Comfort/Sedation Guidelines. Titrate to maintain RASS −3 to −5
   (a) Fentanyl (Sublimaze) IV Bolus 1–2mcg/kg/h (Dilute with 5 ml D5W or NS); IV continuous infusion 1mcg/kg/h (10mcg/ml NS)
   (b) Propofol (Diprivan) IV 10 mg/ml 100 ml; start at 5mcg/kg/min then titrate to SAS 2–3. Use per propofol protocol (not to be used as the sole sedation agent when using a neuromuscular blocker)
   (c) Midazolam (Versed) IV Bolus 2–4 mg IVPush IV Continuous Infusion (2–4 mg/h)
2. Neuro-Muscular blockade (Patient must be ventilated, monitor patient using TOF Micro Stim Device)
   (a) Cisatracurium (Nimbex) IV Bolus 0.1–0.2 mg/kg (1–5 mg/ml D5W or NS) IV Infusion 0.5–10mcg/kg/min (200 mg/200 ml D5W or NS)

   Remember that patient must have Benzodiazepine for amnesia and opiate for neuromuscular pain with a paralytic per hospital policy
3. Shivering
   (a) Buspirone (Buspar) 15 mg PO × 1 ASAP
   (b) Meperidine(Demerol) 25–50 mg IV Q4 h PRN shivering (Limit/avoid use in patients with renal impairment)

   Limit/avoid Demerol use in patients with renal impairment. Demerol (Meperidine) may induce seizure activity in some patients
4. Electrolyte Replacement
   (a) K+, iCa++, Mg++, Phos−− per protocol

5. Hypotension with Normal Ejection Fraction (EF)
   (a) Norepinephrine(Levophed) 8 mg/500NS titrate to MAP >70 mmHg
   (b) NaCl 0.9% titrate to maintain MAP >70 mmHg
6. Hypotension with EF <30 consider: (consult cardiology for use of these meds)
   (a) Dobutamine infusion at 2.5 mcg/kg/min titrate to maintain cardiac index >2.0
   (b) Dopamine at 2.5 mcg/kg/min to maintain MAP >70 mmHG

   Make recommendation for Cardiac output, and SV02 monitoring with therapy
7. Nursing (1:1 ratio for 24 h)
   - Initiate Cooling ASAP (Cool/Warm to 32–34°C) and maintain for 24 h
   - Set device to Max Mode Cooling
   - Inform Respiratory Therapist of Therapy
   - Bed Rest with HOB elevated 30°
   - Vitals: Q15 min during initiation of cooling until therapeutic hypothermia achieved
   - Q 1 h during maintenance phase including shivering assessment
   - Q 15 min for 1 h during initiation of re-warming then Q1 h
   - Neuro checks Q2 h
   - Use Bispectral Index (BIS) monitor to titrate sedation if available (BIS reading between 40 and 60)
   - EKG on admission then Q8 h for 24 h
   - Goal temperature 32–34°C. Call MD if temperature <32°C or if 34°C not achieved within 4 h
   - Consider 500 cc boluses of 4°C IVF if target temperature not achieved in 4 h
   - Ice packs to groin and axilla to achieve target temperature in 4 h; also consider paralytic therapy
   - Electrolyte Replacement Protocol
   - Skin integrity checks per Protocol
   - Oral Care Protocol
   - Insert Salem Sump nasogastric tube, attach to low intermittent suction
   - Insert Foley catheter with temperature probe and attach to cooling device if not available
   - Insert Rectal Temperature probe and attach to cooling device
   - Pressure Ulcer prevention protocol
   - Room temperature should be turned OFF during induction phase
   - Room temperature should be turned back on during re-warming phase (if not already on)
   - Intake and Output hourly
   - Assess for Shivering
   - Daily weights
   - Maintain Arterial Line
   - Maintain Central Venous Lines (Zoll Icy® Cath/Quattro®, 72 h)
   - Maintain target temperature (32–34°C) for 24 h then initiate re-warming
   - Set internal cooling device target temp 37°C set rate to 0.35–0.5°C/h
   - Do not exceed 0.5–1°C/h during re-warming phase
8. Diet/ Nutrition
   (a) NPO×48h
   (b) Level 1 Nutrition Consult
9. Laboratory
   (a) Post arrest
      i. CBC, Chem 10, Base line nutrition lab panel, PT/PTT/INR, DIC panel, Cardiac enzymes, Troponin, ABG, LFT's, Lactate, Ammonia, BNP, Type and Screen, Amylase, Lipase, S-P100 and Pan Culture

   Q4 – 6 h (Refer to guidelines for frequency of labs)
10. Radiology
    (a) Chest X-ray post arrest and QD
11. Cardiology consult
    (a) Consult cardiology in all cases. If cardiac catheterization is indicated, hypothermia should not be delayed.
12. EKG on admission, then Q8 h for 24 h, then QD
13. Echocardiogram
14. Neurology consult
15. Continuous EEG monitoring preferred
16. Respiratory Care
    (a) Ventilator Pressure Control
    (b) Triage Respiratory
    (c) Ventilator Humidifier should be turned OFF and HME should be used during cooling phase

(d) Ventilator Humidifier should be turned ON and HME removed during re-warming phase

17. Skin
18. Please refrain from bathing patients as it may exacerbate shivering. Spot cleaning should be the preferred intervention. Remember shivering causes increased O_2 consumption.

What Data Do I Need?

1. Review patient eligibility, any contraindications, advanced directives and overall prognosis
2. Discuss related issues with health care proxy (Family meeting).
3. Exclude other causes of coma (mass lesions, metabolic coma, seizures etc.)
4. Document baseline neurological evaluation

Equipment List (What Do I Need?)

(All equipment available in CCU in outer closet with key available at the nursing station)

1. Zoll Femoral Line Kit (Icy®/Quattro® Catheter: 4 days, 96 h)
2. Zoll Cool Guard® Machine/XP Thermogard® & Start Up Kit with 500 cc 0.9%NaCL
3. A-line (SVO2) Kit (FloTrac® sensor and Vigileo® Monitoring device)
4. Two 1 l bags of Iced 0.9% NaCL 4°C stored in pharmacy
5. Order Nimbex, Versed, and Fentanyl drips with Iced NaCL
6. Foley temp probe (Rectal temperature probe)
7. Neuromuscular Blockade equipment (TOF Micro Stim Device)
8. Two 18″ gauge peripheral IV sites
9. Two pressure bags (for arterial line and rapid Iced Saline infusion)

What to Do

Note: Data gathering, Monitoring, and Interventions are all initiated immediately and carried simultaneously when feasible

- Cooling procedure
  1. Initiate Sedation with Propofol prior to inducing hypothermia (Versed can be used as alternate to Propofol). Consider paralytic bolus (Nimbex/Vecuronium) to facilitate cooling process. Use Demerol for shivering along with Propofol.
  2. Draw Labs as ordered: Chem10, CBC, PT/PTT/INR, D-Dimer, Fibrinogen, CPK-MB, Troponin, Lactate, Ammonia, Amylase, Lipase, Type and Screen, Pan Cultures, Albumin, Pre Albumin, Transferrin, BNP, ABG, S-P100 and LFT's
  3. Infuse Iced 0.9% NaCl 1–2 l (or 40 ml/kg) over 30 min (peripheral catheter preferred but is not mandatory)
  4. Insert Line and connect Zoll machine and set to maintain temp at 32–34°C
  5. Turn off heat to room and Ventilator (Recommended)
  6. Titrate sedation, and consider using Bair Hugger® and Meperidine (Demerol) for signs of mild to moderate shivering in maintenance phase. (Do not use Bair Hugger® (heat) during Induction)
     - Shivering Scale: Mild Shivering (Facial tremors)
     - Moderate Shivering (Extremity tremors)
     - Severe Shivering (Full body tremors)
  7. Start antibiotics, Ampicillin-Sulbactam (Unasyn) 1.5 g IV now and Q6 h × 3 days then re-assess.
  8. Initiate paralysis with Nimbex only if you are not reaching target temperature within 6 h, or patient experiences moderate to severe shivering on sedation with Meperidine (Demerol), Propofol and Bair Hugger®. Paralysis guided by pupil exam, TOF Micro Stim Device monitor
  9. Also consult Palliative care, Social Services and Life Choice (for Organ Donation) when time permits.
- When therapeutic hypothermia is reached (32–34°C):
  1. Reschedule Unasyn 1.5 g IV Q6 h 72 h from time of first dose (then reassess by chest X-ray for signs of aspiration pneumonia after 72 h)
  2. Chem10, ABG
  3. Maintain sedation, consider Meperidine-(Demerol) and Bair Hugger® to control shivering
  4. If unable to control shivering consider Nimbex gtt with TOF Micro Stim Device monitor (remember an amnesic and analgesic must be used with a paralytic per hospital policy).

- At 4th hour
  1. Chem 10, repeat ABG if needed (treat electrolyte imbalances)
  2. CPK-MB Troponin (Oral Care Protocol should be started)
  3. Unasyn may need to be given (per scheduled dose)
- At 8th hour
  1. Chem 10,
  2. Possible repeat ABG (consider sodium bicarbonate gtt for acidosis)
- At 12th hour
  1. Chem 10, CPK-MB, Troponin
- At 16th hour
  1. Chem 7, ABG if needed
- At 24th hour
  1. CBC, PT/PTT/INR, Chem 10, ABG
  2. Begin re-warming (After 24 h of therapeutic hypothermia 32–34°C)
  3. Set cooling device to 0.35°C/h (controlled rate)
  4. When re-warming is complete maintain patient in Max Mode for possible rebound hyperthermia (Icy® Cath/Quattro® is good for 4 days 96 h)

Note machine will automatically switch to Max Mode after re-warming at no more than 0.5–1°C/h

Basic Maneuvers

- Consider holding paralysis if used and begin sedation holidays as per hospital guidelines
- Other considerations:
  - Resume sedation/paralysis if shivering reoccurs
  - Anticipate relative volume depletion-add fluids as indicated
  - Anticipate possible hypotension
  - Anticipate possible rise in serum K^+
  - Restart HME on ventilator/Turn heat back on in room (if turned off)
  - Anticipate re-cooling if patient seizure activity occurs
- Refer to Seizure guidelines with any seizure activity
- As patient reaches normal (36–37°C) temperature
  - Chem 7, ABG
  - Repeat neurological evaluation while weaning sedation as tolerated
  - CXR – Pneumonia/aspiration is common in this population

(Note: Icy®/Quattro® Catheter is good for 3 days/72 h)

- Daily neurological evaluation, assess for infections/bleeding complications
- Don't forget Life Choice, Palliative care and Social Services consults

Assessment of neurological prognosis (determined 72 h after ROSC)[a]

Brain region	Test 72 h post-ROSC	Specificity for poor outcome	95% CI
Cortical and brainstem	Brain Death Protocol	100%	
Brain stem	Absence of papillary light reflex	100%	88–100%
Cortical	Absence of motor response to pain	100%	93–100%
Cortical	Bilateral absence of early cortical SSEPs	100%	98–100%

[a]Determination of neurological prognosis is unreliable before 72 h after ROSC

[a]Recommended criteria for initiating DNR (do-not-resuscitate) and/or CMO (comfort measures only) *ROSC* return of spontaneous circulation, *SSEP* somatosensory evoked potential

Celsius to Fahrenheit conversion (temperature conversion table)

Celsius	Fahrenheit
38.0	100.4
37.0	98.6
36.0	96.8
35.0	95.0
34.0	93.2
33.0	91.4
32.0	89.6
31.0	87.8
30.0	86.0

Potential laboratory abnormalities associated with hypothermia

Potential lab abnormalities	Treatment
Increased amylase	No intervention unless persistent after re-warming
Abnormal Liver Function Tests	No intervention unless persistent after re-warming
Increased serum glucose	Follow Insulin protocol
Decreased K^+, Mg^{++}, $Phos^{--}$, Ca^{--}	Correct as needed
Increased lactate	Optimize oxygen delivery
Metabolic acidosis	Optimize oxygen delivery
Thrombocytopenia	Correct if <30,000 or to >50,000 if active bleeding
Leukopenia	No intervention unless persistent after re-warming

References

1. Hypothermia after Cardiac Arrest Study Group. Mild therapeutic hypothermia to improve the neurologic outcome after cardiac arrest. N Engl J Med. 2002; 346(8):549–56.
2. Bernard SA, Gray TW, Buist MD, et al. Treatment of comatose survivors of out-of-hospital cardiac arrest with induced hypothermia. N Engl J Med. 2002; 346(8):557–63.
3. ECC Committee, Subcommittees and Task Forces of the American Heart Association. 2005 American Heart Association Guidelines for cardiopulmonary resuscitation and emergency cardiovascular care. Circulation. 2005;112(24 Suppl):V1–203.
4. Nolan JP, Morley PT, Hoek TL, Hickey RW. Therapeutic hypothermia after cardiac arrest. An advisory statement by the Advancement Life support Task Force of the International Liaison committee on Resuscitation. Resuscitation. 2003;57(3):231–5.
5. Haugk M, Sterz F, Grassberger M, et al. Feasibility and efficacy of a new non-invasive surface cooling device in post-resuscitation intensive care medicine. Resuscitation. 2007;75(1):76–81.
6. Hoedemaekers CW, Ezzahti M, Gerritsen A, van der Hoeven JG. Comparison of cooling methods to induce and maintain normo- and hypothermia in intensive care unit patients: a prospective intervention study. Crit Care. 2007;11(4):R91.
7. Holzer M, Mullner M, Sterz F, et al. Efficacy and safety of endovascular cooling after cardiac arrest: cohort study and Bayesian approach. Stroke. 2006; 37(7):1792–7.
8. Lefrant JY, Muller L, de La Coussaye JE, et al. Temperature measurement in intensive care patients: comparison of urinary bladder, oesophageal, rectal, axillary, and inguinal methods versus pulmonary artery core method. Intensive Care Med. 2003;29(3): 414–8.
9. Morris AC, Hay AW, Swann DG, et al. Reducing ventilator-associated pneumonia in intensive care: impact of implementing a care bundle. Crit Care Med. 2011;39(10):2218–24.
10. Schultz MJ, Haas LE. Antibiotics or probiotics as preventive measures against ventilator-associated pneumonia: a literature review. Crit Care. 2011;15(1):R18.
11. Schallom L, Sona C, McSweeney M, Mazuski J. Comparison of forehead and digit oximetry in surgical/trauma patients at risk for decreased peripheral perfusion. Heart Lung. 2007;36(3):188–94.
12. Polderman KH. Application of therapeutic hypothermia in the intensive care unit. Opportunities and pitfalls of a promising treatment modality–part 2: practical aspects and side effects. Intensive Care Med. 2004;30(5):757–69.

8 Complications of Therapeutic Hypothermia Following Cardiac Arrest

Edgar Argulian, Renata Barbosa, Janet Shapiro, and Eyal Herzog

Randomized clinical trials and observational studies have shown that therapeutic hypothermia improves neurologic outcomes and survival in patients following cardiac arrest [1–3]. As the benefit is impressive, with the number needed to treat as low as six patients, therapeutic hypothermia should be applied to more and more patients [4]. At the same time, therapeutic hypothermia is a complex and expensive therapy requiring appropriate equipment, trained personnel, and close patient monitoring. A systematic approach to coordinate care at multiple levels is required for proper patient selection, effective implementation of therapy, and monitoring for possible complications. In our institution, we use a unified pathway-based approach to therapeutic hypothermia [5]. The pathway outlines patient management in a stepwise manner: from the field through the emergency department into the cardiac catheterization laboratory and to the critical care unit (step 1); induced invasive hypothermia protocol in the critical care unit (step 2); and management following the re-warming phase including decisions for future care based on neurologic outcome (step 3). Figure 8.1 shows the pathway for the management of the survivors of out-of-hospital cardiac arrest as implemented at St Luke's Roosevelt Hospital Center, New York. The current chapter focuses on recognition and management of potential complications of hypothermia.

E. Argulian, M.D. (✉) • R. Barbosa, RN •
J. Shapiro, M.D. • E. Herzog, M.D.
Department of Medicine, St. Luke's-Roosevelt Hospital, Columbia University College of Physicians and Surgeons,
New York, NY, USA
e-mail: eargulian@chpnet.org

Choice of the Cooling Method

Several types of cooling methods are available and the particular type is chosen based on institutional preferences [6]. Commercial surface or endovascular cooling devices provide precise temperature control via internal feedback mechanisms, in contrast to the labor-intensive conventional cooling with ice or fans. In our institution, endovascular cooling is used. Endovascular cooling requires central venous access with its potential risks of vascular access complications and infection. Still, it is favored for the following reasons:

1. The target temperature can be rapidly achieved.
2. Precise maintenance of target temperature prevents undercooling and overcooling which may be associated with worse outcomes [7].
3. Re-warming is controlled.
4. Following re-warming, normothermia can be maintained, in order to avoid rebound hyperthermia, especially in infected patients.
5. The central line is always needed for medications.
6. The system allows access to the patient for cardiac interventional and nursing care.

J.B. Lundbye (ed.), *Therapeutic Hypothermia After Cardiac Arrest*,
DOI 10.1007/978-1-4471-2951-6_8,

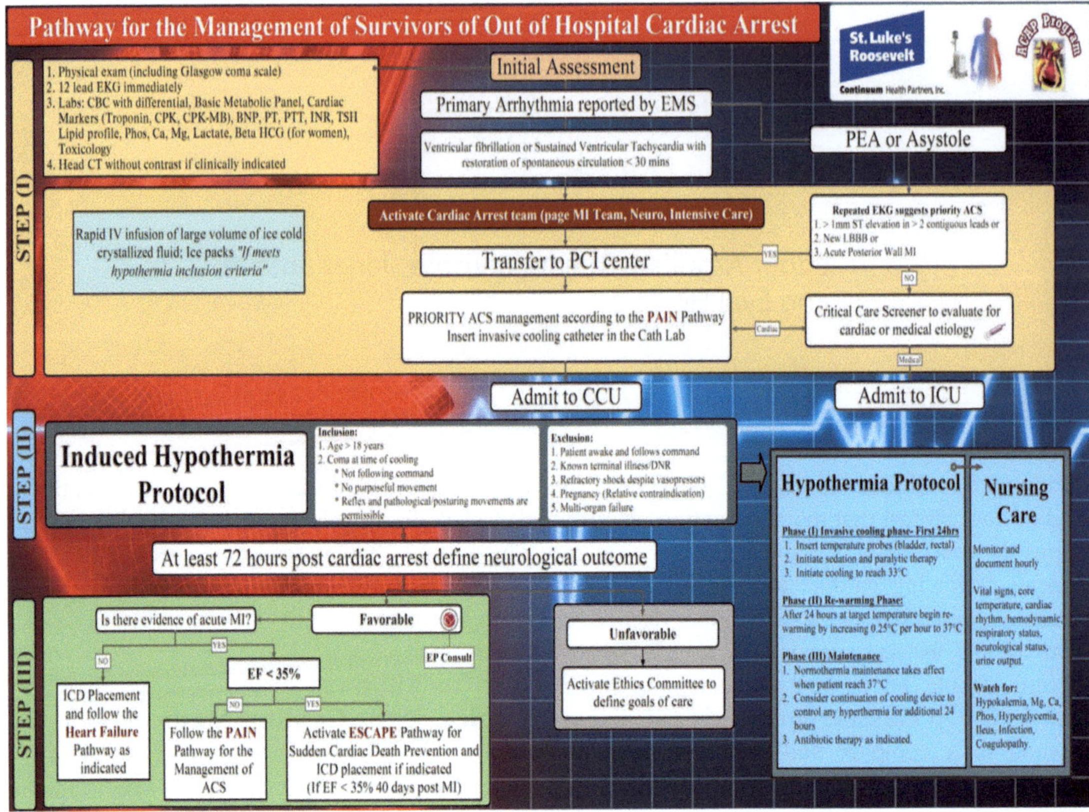

Fig. 8.1 Pathway for the management of out-of-hospital cardiac arrest survivors as implemented at St Luke's Roosevelt Hospital Center, New York

Feasibility studies and observational data suggest a very low rate of complications related to the catheter itself (such as infection, bleeding, or thrombosis) [8, 9].

Physiologic Changes with Therapeutic Hypothermia

While hypothermia <32°C is associated with significant complications, mild therapeutic hypothermia with the target temperature of 32–34°C is well tolerated. The following discussion focuses on the expected physiologic changes with therapeutic hypothermia.

Shivering

Shivering is a major problem during the cooling phase. It is associated with increased metabolic demand and oxygen consumption as well as an increase in the intracranial pressure. Clinical trials used neuromuscular blocking agents to counteract shivering [2, 3]. In fact, many centers commonly use these agents as a part of the initial cooling protocol. During maintenance phase, other pharmacologic agents such as meperidine may be used. Magnesium infusion and local warming maneuvers have also been tried [10]. Generally shivering ceases at the target temperature and patients can be maintained on traditional sedative infusions.

Cardiovascular responses

Cardiovascular responses to cooling include bradycardia, increased peripheral vascular resistance and decreased cardiac output. Despite these changes, organ perfusion is adequate given the decreased metabolic demand. Interestingly, there are reports of favorable outcomes in patients with cardiogenic shock treated with therapeutic hypothermia, probably because the marked decrease in the metabolic needs counteracts the effect of the reduced perfusion [11]. In a hypothermia registry dataset, the incidence of bradycardia (less than 40 beats/min) was reported to be 13% [12]. Bradycardia is usually well tolerated and can potentially decrease the ischemic myocardial burden. It does not need to be treated unless hemodynamically significant.

Hypothermia is commonly associated with QRS complex and QT interval prolongation; one study reported an increased incidence of ventricular premature beats compared to normothermic controls [13]. At the same time, current evidence suggests no increase in the risk of torsades or ventricular fibrillation attributable to mild hypothermia [6]. During re-warming, vasodilation and an increased rate of metabolism are expected; therefore, rapid re-warming may be deleterious [10].

Electrolyte shifts are expected with hypothermia so that frequent protocol-based monitoring of laboratory values is necessary [14]. With cooling, there is intracellular shift of electrolytes and therefore a decrease in the serum concentrations of potassium, magnesium, calcium and phosphate. The decrease in the serum potassium concentration is typically in the range of 1 meq/l [10]. Real-life experience with therapeutic hypothermia shows the incidence of hypokalemia (K<3.0 meq/l) to be 18% [12]. There is evidence that extremes of hypokalemia (K<2.5 meq/l) are associated with an increased risk of arrhythmia in those settings [15]. Although repletion of electrolytes is warranted in the maintenance phase, the clinician must keep in mind that electrolytes will shift during re-warming and serum electrolyte concentrations will increase. The latter finding is usually insignificant but might be a problem in patients with renal impairment. Magnesium repletion during the maintenance phase deserves special attention as repletion can ameliorate shivering and potentially decrease the risk of arrhythmias [10].

Effects on Coagulation

Although deep hypothermia impairs coagulation and possibly inhibits platelet activity, mild hypothermia does not seem to have a clinically significant effect on coagulation and platelet function [10]. Interestingly, hypothermia does not interfere with anti-platelet effect of aspirin but it might attenuate the action of clopidogrel [16, 17].

Metabolic Effects

Decreased carbon dioxide production is attributed to the decreased basal metabolic rate. Arterial blood gas analysis in post-arrest patients frequently shows respiratory acidosis and ventilator settings are set to high minute ventilation. Arterial blood gas analysis should be performed to adjust minute ventilation in order to avoid significant alkalosis [14]. Arterial blood gas analysis itself is affected by temperature. Hypothermia is known to increase pH and decrease PaO_2 and $PaCO_2$ [18]. The practice of correcting arterial blood gas values for temperature is controversial [18, 19].

The metabolic effects of hypothermia also include increased insulin resistance, decreased pancreatic insulin release and increase in counter-insulin hormone production; the sum of these effects results in hyperglycemia in a significant number of patients [10]. Persistent hyperglycemia (>144 mg/dl over 4 h) is strongly associated with adverse outcomes in patients undergoing therapeutic hypothermia [12]. Of note, fingerstick glucose values may be unreliable, showing falsely decreased values due to vasoconstriction [14].

Effects on Drug Metabolism and Risk of Drug Toxicity

Hypothermia affects drug clearance by slowing hepatic enzyme activity. Increased drug levels with hypothermia have been described for benzodiazepines, propofol, anticonvulsants, and neuromuscular blocking agents [20]. At the same time, pharmacodynamic effects of medications might be attenuated, thereby counterbalancing the increase in the serum levels. The re-warming phase deserves particular attention because pharmacokinetic and pharmacodynamic effects are reversed, now potentially predisposing to significant drug toxicity [21].

Immune System Effects

Hypothermia is associated with neutropenia and possibly suppression of immune responses such as inflammatory cytokine production [22, 23]. Those effects may contribute to increased susceptibility to infection as discussed below.

Complications of Hypothermia

Most complications follow from the physiologic changes discussed above.

Cardiovascular Complications

Overall arrhythmic risk is high in patients undergoing hypothermia following cardiac arrest, but it does not seem to differ significantly from those patients who do not receive therapeutic hypothermia [6]. In patients who have cardiac arrest *during* therapeutic hypothermia, standard ACLS protocol should be followed [10]. Defibrillation threshold might be higher with hypothermia but this usually applies to moderate to severe hypothermia [16]. Rapid re-warming may potentiate hemodynamic instability and should be avoided.

Bleeding Complications

The risk of bleeding requiring blood transfusion was reported in 4% of a large registry of hypothermia patients [12]. This risk is substantially increased by percutaneous interventions such as coronary interventions and intra-aortic balloon placement [12]. At the same time, there is evidence that those interventions might improve survival in post-cardiac arrest patients and they should *not* be withheld if clinically necessary [24]. Bleeding complications are not associated with increased mortality or worsening neurologic outcomes in patients treated with therapeutic hypothermia [12].

Infection

Infectious complications, especially pneumonia are common after cardiac arrest [12]. In a retrospective database review of 537 post-cardiac arrest patients in whom the majority underwent therapeutic hypothermia, infectious complications were frequent. The most common infections were pneumonia, followed by bloodstream and catheter infection. Although infections were associated with increased duration of mechanical ventilation and intensive care unit length of stay, there was no impact on mortality or on neurologic outcomes [25]. A recent study from this database demonstrated an increased risk of development of early (within 3 days) pneumonia, associated with longer mechanical ventilation and intensive care unit stay but no impact on intensive care unit mortality [26]. Recognition of infection is a challenge in patients undergoing hypothermia as fever will not be seen. Clinicians should have a low threshold for initiating antibiotic therapy when infection is suspected (e.g., leukocytosis, unexplained pulmonary infiltrates) [10, 27].

Seizures

Seizures may occur following cardiac arrest due to the ischemic cerebral injury. Seizures do not occur more commonly in patients with therapeutic hypothermia but they may be associated with adverse outcomes. In a study by Nielsen et al. mortality rate exceeded 80% in patients with seizures requiring anticonvulsants [12]. At the same time, use of neuromuscular blocking agents can mask seizure activity in those patients and continuous EEG monitoring may be required for patient monitoring [10]. If seizures are diagnosed, they are aggressively managed with intravenous anticonvulsants.

Challenges in Nursing Needs for the Patient Related to Hypothermia

There are many challenges for the nurse when caring for a patient undergoing therapeutic hypothermia during all phases of therapy. Some of the specific aspects of nursing care are outlined below.

Skin Breakdown

Patients on therapeutic hypothermia are strongly predisposed to skin breakdown due to immobility with deep sedation and therapeutic paralysis during the cooling period, hypotension and skin hypoperfusion due to peripheral vasoconstriction. Therefore, meticulous skin care is of paramount importance. Routine care includes frequent patient positioning (every 2 h) and skin inspection. We recommend pressure reducing products such as overlays and heel protectors. The use of special mattresses that have favorable pressure redistribution surface and low air loss is limited by cost and availability but it should also be considered.

Maintenance of Intravenous Lines

Stable intravenous access is necessary for patients undergoing therapeutic hypothermia. Patients will have multiple blood samples drawn at frequent intervals. They also receive multiple medications including intravenous infusions. At the same time, intravenous lines may serve as ports of infection. Therefore, lines and their respective sites should be monitored routinely for signs of infection and infiltration and routinely changed based on institutional infection control protocols.

Prevention of Ventilator-Associated Pneumonia

Patients on the hypothermia protocol have a high incidence of pneumonia as discussed earlier. Recognition of pneumonia may be difficult due to absence of fever and blunted inflammatory response. The change in quantity and quality of respiratory secretions may help in timely recognition of infection. The prevention of ventilator-associated pneumonia is essential. Measures include elevation of the head of the bed to 30–45°. Oral care and oropharyngeal cleaning and decontamination with an antiseptic agent are also practiced routinely at our institution. General infection control guidelines and strict adherence to hand washing and sterile technique for procedures must be followed.

Gastrointestinal Issues

Gastric motility and absorption are reduced during hypothermia. Feeding is generally avoided during the induction and maintenance phases. Once feeding is started in the re-warming phase residuals and motility should be assessed. Early administration of a bowel regimen such as stool softeners, soluble fiber, and laxatives are important in attempting to maintain function.

Neurological Assessment

Neurological assessment is extremely important for patients undergoing the hypothermia protocol. As seizures are significant sequelae of the cerebral injury and must be identified and treated immediately, the nurse must be vigilant in looking for any sign of subtle seizures such as blinking and twitching. Using a sedation scale and protocol is valuable with hourly monitoring of sedation. The initial goal is deep sedation during the cooling and re-warming stages; then the sedation should be reduced or stopped in order to assess the mental status. A thorough neurological assessment includes assessment of level of consciousness, pupil reaction, and motor responses.

Preventive Measures

For gastric stress ulcer prophylaxis, we typically employ proton pump inhibitors or H2 receptor blockers. We do not routinely use antacids for stress ulcer prophylaxis. Deep venous thrombosis prophylaxis should be provided to all patients undergoing therapeutic hypothermia. Pharmacologic prophylaxis with heparin is generally the preferred modality.

Family Support

Because of the unexpected nature and uncertain course of a patient who survives a cardiac arrest, family support and education are very important. Families are often overwhelmed when dealing with the fact that their loved one is critically ill, in need of intensive care and life support. In attempting to decrease family anxiety, nurses should explain the purpose of hypothermia therapy, the equipment involved, procedures, and monitoring. The nurse should also reassure the family that comfort to the patient is being provided and that sedation and analgesia are being appropriately utilized. Even though prognosis is uncertain the nurse should maintain an informative and open rapport with the family.

Conclusion

Therapeutic hypothermia is a beneficial therapy which improves survival and neurologic outcomes in survivors of cardiac arrest. The many effects of hypothermia on organ systems pose potential complications. Clinicians, both physicians and nurses, must anticipate these potential complications. A structured approach to the process of providing hypothermia involves the recognition and treatment of these complications.

References

1. Arrich J, Holzer M, Herkner H, Mullner M. Cochrane corner: hypothermia for neuroprotection in adults after cardiopulmonary resuscitation. Anesth Analg. 2010;110:1239.
2. Hypothermia after Cardiac Arrest Study Group. Mild therapeutic hypothermia to improve the neurologic outcome after cardiac arrest. N Engl J Med. 2002; 346:549–56.
3. Bernard SA, Gray TW, Buist MD, et al. Treatment of comatose survivors of out-of-hospital cardiac arrest with induced hypothermia. N Engl J Med. 2002; 346:557–63.
4. Holzer M, Bernard SA, Hachimi-Idrissi S, Roine RO, Sterz F, Mullner M. Hypothermia for neuroprotection after cardiac arrest: systematic review and individual patient data meta-analysis. Crit Care Med. 2005; 33:414–8.
5. Herzog E, Shapiro J, Aziz EF, et al. Pathway for the management of survivors of out-of-hospital cardiac arrest. Crit Pathw Cardiol. 2010;9:49–54.
6. Holzer M. Targeted temperature management for comatose survivors of cardiac arrest. N Engl J Med. 2010;363:1256–64.
7. Merchant RM, Abella BS, Peberdy MA, et al. Therapeutic hypothermia after cardiac arrest: unintentional overcooling is common using ice packs and conventional cooling blankets. Crit Care Med. 2006;34:S490–4.
8. Holzer M, Mullner M, Sterz F, et al. Efficacy and safety of endovascular cooling after cardiac arrest: cohort study and Bayesian approach. Stroke. 2006; 37:1792–7.
9. Al-Senani FM, Graffagnino C, Grotta JC, et al. A prospective, multicenter pilot study to evaluate the feasibility and safety of using the CoolGard System and Icy catheter following cardiac arrest. Resuscitation. 2004;62:143–50.
10. Seder DB, Jarrah S. Therapeutic hypothermia for cardiac arrest: a practical approach. Curr Neurol Neurosci Rep. 2008;8:508–17.
11. Skulec R, Kovarnik T, Dostalova G, Kolar J, Linhart A. Induction of mild hypothermia in cardiac arrest survivors presenting with cardiogenic shock syndrome. Acta Anaesthesiol Scand. 2008;52:188–94.
12. Nielsen N, Hovdenes J, Nilsson F, et al. Outcome, timing and adverse events in therapeutic hypothermia after out-of-hospital cardiac arrest. Acta Anaesthesiol Scand. 2009;53:926–34.
13. Tiainen M, Parikka HJ, Makijarvi MA, Takkunen OS, Sarna SJ, Roine RO. Arrhythmias and heart rate variability during and after therapeutic hypothermia for cardiac arrest. Crit Care Med. 2009;37: 403–9.
14. Kupchik NL. Development and implementation of a therapeutic hypothermia protocol. Crit Care Med. 2009;37:S279–84.
15. Mirzoyev SA, McLeod CJ, Bunch TJ, Bell MR, White RD. Hypokalemia during the cooling phase of therapeutic hypothermia and its impact on arrhythmogenesis. Resuscitation. 2010;81:1632–6.
16. Arpino PA, Greer DM. Practical pharmacologic aspects of therapeutic hypothermia after cardiac arrest. Pharmacotherapy. 2008;28:102–11.
17. Bjelland TW, Hjertner O, Klepstad P, Kaisen K, Dale O, Haugen BO. Antiplatelet effect of clopidogrel is reduced in patients treated with therapeutic hypothermia after cardiac arrest. Resuscitation. 2010;81: 1627–31.
18. Shapiro BA. Temperature correction of blood gas values. Respir Care Clin N Am. 1995;1:69–76.
19. Bacher A. Effects of body temperature on blood gases. Intensive Care Med. 2005;31:24–7.
20. Tortorici MA, Kochanek PM, Poloyac SM. Effects of hypothermia on drug disposition, metabolism, and response: a focus of hypothermia-mediated alterations on the cytochrome P450 enzyme system. Crit Care Med. 2007;35:2196–204.
21. Janata A, Holzer M. Hypothermia after cardiac arrest. Prog Cardiovasc Dis. 2009;52:168–79.
22. Polderman KH. Mechanisms of action, physiological effects, and complications of hypothermia. Crit Care Med. 2009;37:S186–202.
23. Kimura A, Sakurada S, Ohkuni H, Todome Y, Kurata K. Moderate hypothermia delays proinflammatory cytokine

production of human peripheral blood mononuclear cells. Crit Care Med. 2002;30:1499–502.

24. Sunde K, Soreide E. Therapeutic hypothermia after cardiac arrest: where are we now? Curr Opin Crit Care. 2011;17:247–53.
25. Mongardon N, Perbet S, Lemiale V, et al. Infectious complications in out-of-hospital cardiac arrest patients in the therapeutic hypothermia era. Crit Care Med. 2011;39:1359–64.
26. Perbet S, Mongardon N, Dumas F, et al. Early onset pneumonia after cardiac arrest: characteristics, risk factors and influence on prognosis. Am J Respir Crit Care Med. 2011;184:1048–54.
27. Acquarolo A, Urli T, Perone G, Giannotti C, Candiani A, Latronico N. Antibiotic prophylaxis of early onset pneumonia in critically ill comatose patients. A randomized study. Intensive Care Med. 2005;31:510–6.

Pharmacology and Therapeutic Hypothermia

9

William L. Baker

Introduction

Various randomized clinical trials have demonstrated the beneficial effects of therapeutic hypothermia on survival and neurological function following cardiac arrest [1–4]. Despite these well-documented outcomes, a number of physiologic and metabolic complications have been identified [see Chap. 8] [5]. More specifically, data examining the impact of reducing patients' core body temperature to 32–34°C on drug disposition and therapeutic response remains incomplete [6–8]. Given the number of pharmacologic agents provided to patients following cardiac arrest, knowledge of the impact of therapeutic hypothermia on their pharmacokinetic, pharmacodynamic, efficacy and safety parameters is paramount. This chapter includes an in-depth review of both animal and human data as well as provides recommendations for clinical use for pharmacologic agents routinely used in the management of patients undergoing therapeutic hypothermia following cardiac arrest.

W.L. Baker, Pharm.D., BCPS
Department of Pharmacy and Medicine, University of Connecticut, Schools of Pharmacy and Medicine, Storrs, Farmington, CT, USA
e-mail: wbaker@uchc.edu

Effects of Hypothermia on Drug Disposition

A large proportion of pharmacologic agents administered to patients following cardiac arrest are hepatically metabolized by the cytochrome P450 (CYP) enzyme system [6, 8]. Alterations in enzymatic activity and proficiency can affect the serum concentrations of these drugs and potentially their beneficial or harmful effects [9, 10]. A study by Fritz and colleagues utilized a juvenile swine model to examine the effects of therapeutic hypothermia on hepatic microsomal CYP3A4 activity [11]. This investigations showed the temperature dependency of CYP3A4 with a 69% (± 1%) reduction in activity seen at 32°C compared with a normothermic control (38°C; $p<0.05$). The reasons behind this reduced CYP450 enzymatic activity during hypothermia are unclear. Some theories include a reduced affinity of CYP450 for specific substrates, a decreased rate of redox reactions performed by CYP450 enzymes, amongst others [6]. Tortorici and colleagues proposed an enzymatic timeline of hypothermia-associated changes in CYP450-mediated activity [6]. During the cooling process, CYP450 activity is significantly reduced with a return to normal activity after rewarming. Additional studies are required to better elucidate the relationship between reduced core temperatures and cytochromal enzyme activity and metabolic capacity.

J.B. Lundbye (ed.), *Therapeutic Hypothermia After Cardiac Arrest*,
DOI 10.1007/978-1-4471-2951-6_9,

Sedatives and Neuromuscular Blockers

Propofol

Propofol is a general anesthetic agent that has a rapid onset and short duration of action [12–14]. General critical care medicine guidelines recommend its use in clinical situations requiring rapid awakening for either neurologic or respiratory assessment [15]. It is given via a continuous intravenous infusion at rates commonly ranging from 5–80 mcg/kg/min. Propofol is a high extraction drug whose clearance is highly dependent on hepatic blood flow [12–14]. Thus, reductions in hepatic blood flow during therapeutic hypothermia may alter systemic propofol concentrations resulting in deeper sedation states and increased risk for adverse events [16, 17].

A single published study has evaluated the impact of hypothermia on the disposition of propofol (Table 9.1) [16]. Leslie and colleagues enrolled six healthy volunteers and randomized them to have their core temperature reduced on 1 day and normothermia maintained on the other [16]. Patients were intubated with anesthesia initiated using thiopental and isoflurane. They were then cooled using leg cooling, reaching a core temperature of 34.6°C while on the other day the core temperature was maintained at 37.0°C. Once the target temperature was achieved, a bolus of propofol 1 mg/kg followed by a continuous infusion at 5 mg/kg/h and continued for 4 h. Blood samples were taken throughout this timeframe to determine propofol blood concentrations. The authors showed that reducing patients' core body temperature to a mean of 34.0±0.01°C resulted in a 28% increase in propofol blood concentrations compared with those maintained at 37.0±0.01°C ($p<0.05$) with the greatest difference seen in the first 5 min of the infusion (Fig. 9.1) [16].

Benzodiazepines

This class of medications is used for their sedative and hypnotic properties and is frequently utilized in critically ill patients [15]. The agents most commonly prescribed include midazolam, lorazepam, and diazepam. Midazolam and lorazepam are administered as continuous intravenous infusions at common doses ranging from 0.04 to 0.2 mg/kg/h and 0.01 to 0.1 mg/kg/h, respectively [15]. The only agent in this class that has been studied during therapeutic hypothermia is midazolam which has a rapid onset and short duration of action [18–20]. It is highly dependent on hepatic metabolism, primarily through CYP3A4 and has an active metabolite, alpha-hydroxymidazolam, that can accumulate and prolong its sedative effect [21, 22]. A recent systematic review of therapeutic hypothermia protocols reported that midazolam was the sedative of choice in 57% of the institutions studied [23].

Two published studies has evaluated the impact of hypothermia on the disposition of midazolam [18, 19]. Fukuoka and colleagues enrolled 15 brain-injury patients receiving continuous infusions of midazolam (5 mcg/kg/min) for maintenance of their sedation [18]. Eight patients underwent hypothermia within 3–4 h of sustaining their injury to a target core body temperature of 32–24°C while the other seven were maintained at 36–37.5°C. The authors showed a sustained increase in serum midazolam concentrations in patients undergoing hypothermia with a sharp decline following the core body temperature rising beyond 35°C. The normothermic patients saw a plateau in their serum midazolam concentrations following an initial mild rise. Unfortunately, statistical comparisons between the hypothermic and normothermic groups were not performed. However, significant differences in a few pharmacokinetic parameters (volume of distribution, elimination rate constant, and clearance) were seen in the "cooling" states versus "rewarming" stages of the hypothermic group. The second study by Hostler and colleagues conducted a prospective, randomized, controlled study of six healthy male volunteers [19]. Patients were randomized to one of four groups: (1) Warm saline (37.0°C); (2) warm saline (37.0°C)+magnesium; (3) cold saline (4.0°C); (4) cold saline (4.0°C)+magnesium. All groups received three

Table 9.1 Select human studies evaluating effect of therapeutic hypothermia on drug disposition

References	Drug	Pts. (n)	Population	Dosage	Target temperature	Pharmacokinetic alterations (versus normothermia)
Leslie et al. [16]	Propofol	6	Healthy volunteers	1 mg/kg IV bolus, 5 mg/kg/h IV infusion	34.02°C vs. 36.6°C	↑ Serum concentrations by 28% vs. normothermia ($p<0.05$)
	Atracurium			0.5 mg/kg IV bolus		↑ Duration of action vs. normothermia
Fukuoka et al. [18]	Midazolam	15	Brain injury	5 mcg/kg/min IV infusion	32–24°C vs. 36–37.5°C	↑ Serum concentrations during hypothermia vs. normothermia
Hostler et al. [19]	Midazolam	6	Healthy volunteers	2 mg IV q10 min × 3 doses	35.4–35.8°C vs. 37°C	No differences in half-life, C_{max}, or $AUC_{0\text{-inf}}$, ↓ midazolam clearance during hypothermia
Heier et al. [33]	Vecuronium	10	Elective surgery	0.1 mg/kg IV bolus	34.7°C vs. 36.5°C	↑ Duration of action & spontaneous recovery time vs. normothermia
Heier et al. [34]	Vecuronium	10	Elective surgery	3 mcg/kg/min IV infusion × 10 min	34.4°C vs. 36.8°C	No differences in pharmacodynamic variables (C_{ss50}, K_{eo})
Caldwell et al. [35]	Vecuronium	12	Healthy volunteers	5 mcg/kg/min IV infusion	<35.0°C vs. 35.0–35.9°C vs. 36.0–36.9°C vs. >37.0°C	↑ Duration of action with ↓ core temperature. Cl ↓ by 13% for every °C ↓ in temperature
Russell et al. [53]	Remifentanil	16	Cardiac bypass surgery	2–5 mcg/kg IV bolus	28–30°C vs. >35–36°C	↓ Clearance by 20% vs. normothermia
Michelsen et al. [54]	Remifentanil	68	Cardiac bypass surgery	1–3 mcg/kg/min IV infusion	<28°C vs. 28–32°C vs. 32–27°C	↓ Clearance by 6.37% with each degree (Celsius) ↓ in temperature below 37°C
Bjelland et al. [66]	Clopidogrel	25	Post-cardiac arrest	300–600 mg PO bolus, 75 mg/day	33–34°C	100% clopidogrel resistance at 24 h & 70% resistance on day 3
McAllister et al. [70]	Propranolol	12	Cardiac bypass surgery	40–320 mg/day prior to surgery	26°C vs. 37°C	↑ Serum concentrations, ↓ volume of distribution & total body clearance vs. normothermia

Cl clearance, C_{ss50} plasma concentration producing 50% decrease in adductor pollicis twitch tension, *IV* intravenous, K_{eo} rate constant for equilibrium of vecuronium between plasma and the neuromuscular junction, *n* number, *NR* not reported, *PO* orally, *pts* patients

doses of midazolam 2 mg each 10-min apart with blood samples routinely drawn to determine serum midazolam concentrations. No differences in half-life, C_{max}, or $AUC_{0\text{-inf}}$ were seen between the normothermic and hypothermic groups. However, a significant decrease in midazolam clearance was seen in the hypothermic groups versus the normothermic groups. In fact, the authors suggested that clearance could be decreased by 11.1% for every degree the core body temperature is reduced below 36.5°C.

Neuromuscular Blockers

Neuromuscular blockers (NMBs) are a heterogenous group of pharmacologic agents that are frequently used to induce therapeutic hypothermia

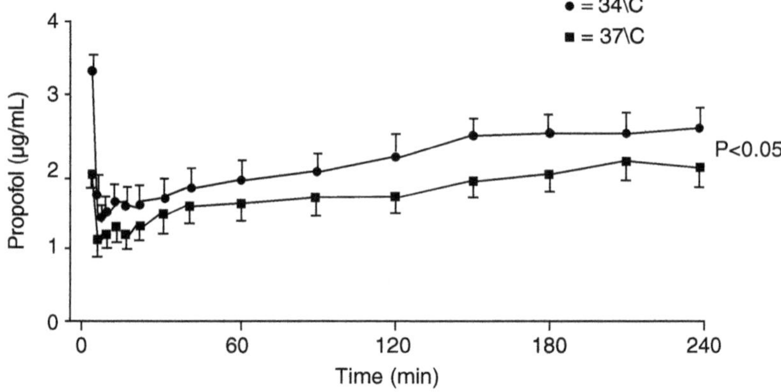

Fig. 9.1 Impact of hypothermia on serum propofol concentrations (Modified from Ref. [16]

as well as prevent severe shivering during the procedure [2, 3, 24–26]. Agents within this class are classified as either depolarizing or nondepolarizing drugs. The only available depolarizing NMB is currently succinylcholine, which does not have any data for use during therapeutic hypothermia. The more commonly used nondepolarizing NMBs include agents such as pancuronium, rocuronium, and cisatracurium, among others [27]. Clinical monitoring for efficacy with NMBs is performed using peripheral nerve stimulators and the "train of four" method, which has been described in detail elsewhere [27, 28]. However, the twitch response elicited during nerve stimulation may be altered during therapeutic hypothermia and may not represent the optimal modality for monitoring NMBs [29]. Moreover, data suggest the duration and depth of blockade may be appreciably affected during hypothermia necessitating closer clinical monitoring [29]. Thus, an in-depth knowledge of the clinical data is imperative for practitioners using NMBs during therapeutic hypothermia.

Three studies were identified using various animal models to determine the impact of hypothermia on the pharmacokinetics, pharmacodynamics, and clinical actions of NMBs [30–32]. The first evaluated the impact of decreasing core body temperature to either 29°C or 34°C versus 39°C in 14 cats receiving pancuronium [30]. Although no differences were seen between the 34°C and 39°C groups, the duration of block was approximately three times longer in the 29°C, which also had a plasma half-life of 46 min versus 21–25 min in the other groups. It was hypothesized that these pharmacodynamic changes were the result of delayed biliary and urinary excretion of pancuronium in conjunction with an increased sensitivity to the block [30]. A subsequently published rat model evaluated four nondepolaring NMBs, d-tubocurarine, pancuronium, metocurine, and gallamine, at temperatures of 25°C, 31°C, and 37°C [10]. Although a two-fold increase in ED_{50} (drug concentration producing a twitch ratio of 0.50 for the temperature studied) was seen for three of the four agents, only pancuronium had efficacy that was unaffected by temperature. This suggests that larger doses of three NMBs would be required to get the desired effect, whereas no changes in pancuronium were seen [31]. Lastly, another rat liver model showed that hypothermia (28°C) significantly reduced hepatic uptake of the NMB vecuronium, decreasing its metabolism and significantly increasing tissue concentrations compared with normothermia (38°C) [32]. Thus, it appears that differing effects of hypothermia are seen depending on the particular animal model used which makes need and interpretation of human data more critical to clinical decision makers.

A total of five studies enrolling human subjects have been published, evaluating use of various NMBs at decreased temperatures [16, 33–35]. Vecuronium has been evaluated in three of these studies [33–35], while the fourth evaluated atracurium [16]. In both healthy volunteers as well as elective surgical populations, decreasing core

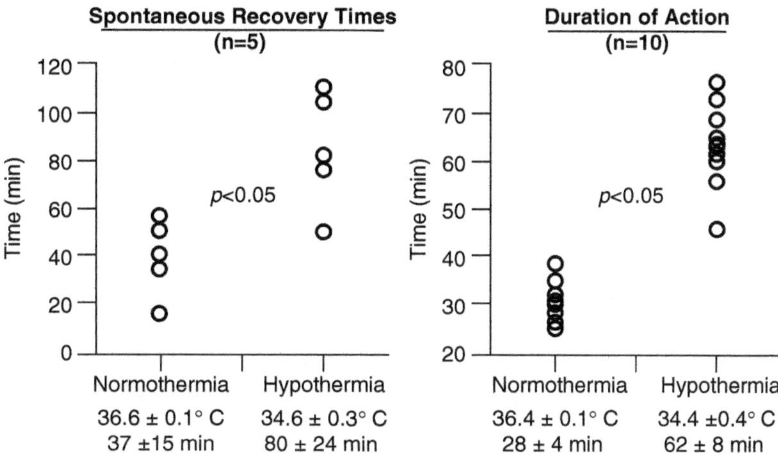

Fig. 9.2 Hypothermia increases duration of action & spontaneous recovery of vecuronium blockade (Modified from Ref. [33])

body temperature consistently increased the duration of action of blockade with vecuronium as well as increased spontaneous recovery time (Fig. 9.2) [33]. In order to identify the mechanism behind these changes, Heier and colleagues studied the pharmacodynamic changes seen with vecuronium during mild intraoperative hypothermia [34]. They hypothesized that hypothermia induced an increase in neuromuscular junction sensitivity resulting in a decreased rate of equilibrium between the junction and the plasma. Interestingly, they saw no significant changed in a number of pharmacodynamic variables suggesting that a concentration-effect is unlikely the explanation for the prolonged blockade seen with vecuronium during hypothermia [34]. Alterations in the drugs distribution and elimination may be the rationale. In fact, Caldwell and colleagues showed that for every 1°C reduction in core body temperature, a decrease in vecuronium clearance of 13% is seen [35]. Thus, it seems reasonable that dosing requirements may be altered in patients undergoing therapeutic hypothermia. A study by Cammu and colleagues of 17 patients during hypothermic cardiopulmonary bypass suggested that although dosing requirements of the NMB rocuronium were not altered, the infusion rates for cisatracurium should be halved during hypothermia [36]. Prior investigations in patients undergoing hypothermic cardiopulmonary bypass have shown similar results to both healthy volunteers and those having elective surgery without bypass [37–41].

Summary

Current practice guidelines recommend use of sedation, including benzodiazepines and propofol, during the process of therapeutic hypothermia to prevent shivering and achieve target core body temperatures [25, 26]. One of the guidelines specifies that midazolam or propofol can be used with no preference given between the two. Interestingly, a systematic review of 44 studies evaluating anesthesia and analgesia protocols in 68 intensive care units (ICUs) during therapeutic hypothermia following cardiac arrest showed that midazolam was preferred in 57% of ICUs whereas propofol was preferred in 19% of ICUs [23]. Since previous studies have shown that the clinical effects of both these agents can be increased during hypothermia, factors such as the patients comorbidities and local practice patterns should dictate sedative use. Following initiation, clearly specified sedation goals should be provided and monitored on an ongoing basis. Additionally, common adverse events (both clinical and laboratory) should be closely followed during cooldown, maintenance, and warm-up periods of therapeutic hypothermia. If shivering becomes an issue in the patients and NMB use is required, guidelines recommend that rocuronium or cisatracurium are reasonable options [25, 26]. Patients should receive continuous electroencephalographic monitoring during sustained neuromuscular blockade, remembering that the duration of action is prolonged during cooling.

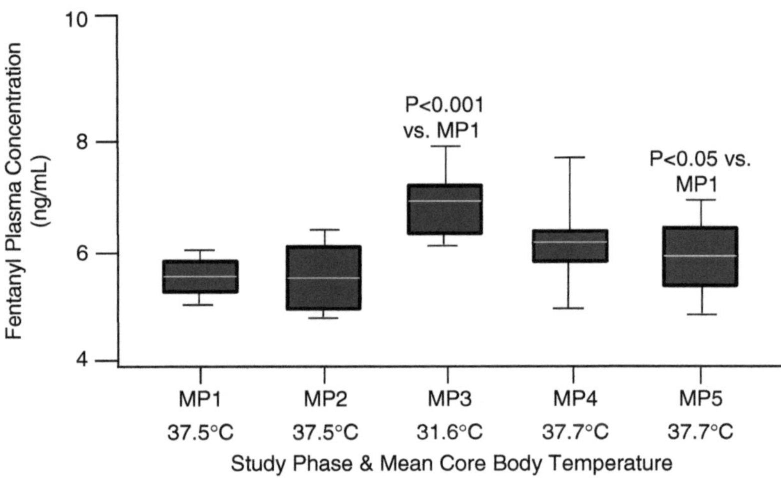

Fig. 9.3 Effects of hypothermia on plasma fentanyl concentrations in a swine model (Modified from Ref. [45])

Anesthetics

Fentanyl/Remifentanil

Fentanyl is a synthetic opioid analgesic recommended for use in critically ill patients requiring intravenous pain relief, particularly those with hemodynamic instability or renal impairment [15]. It is primarily metabolized hepatically by the CYP3A4 isoenzyme to inactive metabolites [15, 42]. Because it is the most frequently used anesthetic in institutions providing therapeutic hypothermia following cardiac arrest, the impact of reduced body temperatures on its pharmacologic actions are relevant to practicing clinicians [23].

A number of experimental animal and human models have evaluated the impact of hypothermia on fentanyl pharmacokinetics in different populations [43–50]. Four of these studies evaluated various animal models, including rats and pigs [43–47]. The animal models all showed significant increases in serum fentanyl concentrations during periods of cooling. Fritz and colleagues showed a 25±11% increase in plasma fentanyl concentrations during hypothermia (31.6°C±0.2°C) versus normothermia (37.7°C±0.3°C) which remained elevated for 6 h following rewarming in a study of seven juvenile pigs (Fig. 9.3) [45]. A more recent study of 32 adult Sprague-Dawley rats showed that mild hypothermia (33°C) significantly decreased the systemic clearance of fentanyl after cardiac arrest versus normothermia (37°C) (61.5±11.5–48.9±8.95 mL/kg/min; $p<0.05$) (Fig. 9.4) [46]. The authors hypothesized that these alterations were due to reductions in hepatic cytochromal P450 3A4 metabolic capacity during the hypothermic state. Interestingly, the brain penetration of fentanyl was not significantly altered during hypothermia suggesting that reductions in infusion rates to combat the elevated serum levels might result in lower brain levels and a reduced therapeutic effect [46]. This theory requires additional study in human patients to confirm these findings.

The currently available human studies evaluate the use of fentanyl during cardiopulmonary bypass in either adult or pediatric populations undergoing cardiac surgery which target core body temperatures from <32°C to 34°C [43, 48–50]. During the periods of cooling in patients receiving cardiopulmonary bypass, some studies have shown both significant increases in serum fentanyl concentrations as well as the elimination phase half-life of fentanyl [47, 49]. Others have not demonstrated significant differences in plasma fentanyl concentrations during cardiopulmonary bypass, particularly when fentanyl was given via a continuous infusion [48, 50]. Overall, the human data has not routinely supported the findings from animal studies, although the designs and populations differ considerably. Until more studies become available in human populations, particularly those following cardiac arrest, clinicians should anticipate elevated fentanyl concentrations and prolonged effects during and

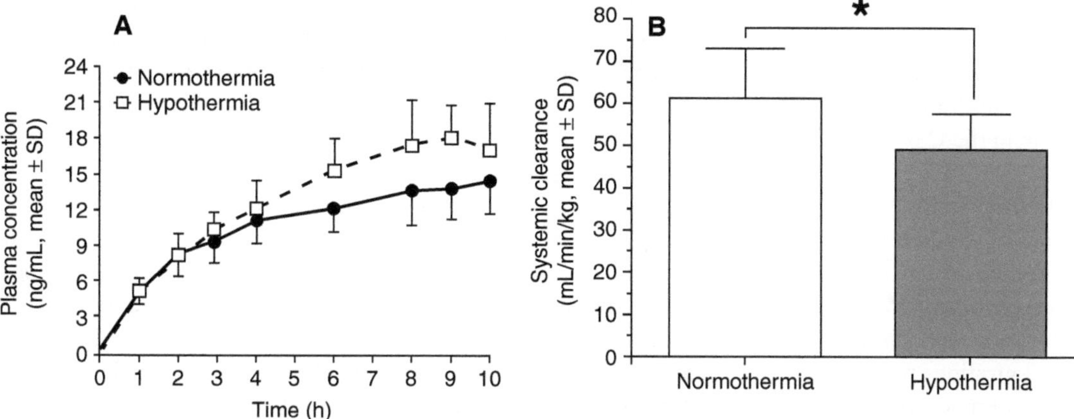

Fig. 9.4 (**a**) Shows that the fentanyl plasma time-concentration profile was elevated under hypothermic conditions. (**b**) Shows that hypothermia resulted in a modest decrease in the systemic clearance of fentanyl. * $p < 0.05$. Fentanyl concentrations & systemic clearance in 32 Sprague-Dawley rats following cardiac arrest (Reprinted with permission from Ref. [46])

after therapeutic hypothermia with appropriate monitoring for effect and adverse events.

Remifentanil is a potent, short-acting derivative of fentanyl that has been increasingly used during therapeutic hypothermia following cardiac arrest [15, 51]. Due to its short duration of action (half-life 10–20 min), it is often provided as an intravenous continuous infusion. Remifentanil also undergoes N-dealkylation by CYP450 isoenzymes to some degree, alterations to which could affect its plasma concentrations during therapeutic hypothermia [52]. Two studies of the effect of hypothermia during cardiopulmonary bypass on remifentanil pharmacokinetics were identified [53, 54]. Russell and colleagues administered either remifentanil 2 or 5 mcg/kg intravenous boluses for three doses in 16 patients undergoing coronary revascularization with cardiopulmonary bypass [53]. During bypass, patients had their core body temperature reduced to 28–30°C then increased to >36°C after that. Clearance of remifentanil was reduced by 20% during hypothermia compared with normothermia, regardless of the dose administered (ANOVA; $p=0.0057$). The authors attributed this effect to a reduced hydrolytic enzyme activity during lower body temperature states [53]. The second study was a randomized, open-label, parallel group trial of 68 patients undergoing coronary artery bypass graft surgery that assigned patients to receive remifentanil infusions of 1, 2, or 3 mcg/kg/min [54]. They found similar results to those of Russell and colleagues [14], demonstrating a 6.37% (such as increase, decrease, change) in remifentanil clearance with each degree Celsius decrease in temperature below 37°C. Interestingly, the authors suggest that consistent blood levels of remifentanil may be reached if the continuous infusion rate is decreased by approximately 30% for every 5°C decrease in the patient's core body temperature [54]. This is one of the only clinical studies that provides a dosing algorithm based on pharmacokinetic alterations during therapeutic hypothermia.

Morphine

Morphine is another opioid analgesic that is metabolized to two active metabolites, all of which accumulate with renal dysfunction [55]. As compared with fentanyl, relatively few institutions have morphine as their standard analgesic for use during therapeutic hypothermia [23]. Two animal studies and a single human study evaluating the impact of hypothermia on the disposition of morphine were found [55–57]. Puig and colleagues showed that the potency of morphine was significantly decreased at 30°C compared with 37°C [55]. The second animal study used a canine model to show that the levels of morphine in the cerebral spinal fluid (CSF) were significantly increased at a core body temperature of 30°C compared with 37°C ($p<0.05$) [56]. They also saw a prolonged elimination half-life of morphine in the CSF at 30°C (3.6 ± 0.8 h) compared with 37°C (1.5 ± 0.17 h; $p<0.05$). The only available human study evaluated the impact of prolonged hypothermia on the pharmacokinetics of morphine in ten infants with hypoxic ischemic encephalopathy [57]. They showed that morphine clearance was significantly reduced and serum concentrations were significantly increased in the infants randomized to hypothermia (mean rectal temperature 33.4°C) versus the normothermic control group (mean rectal temperature 36.7°C). Taken together, these studies suggest that serum levels, as well as duration of effect, of morphine during therapeutic hypothermia are likely to be elevated, potentially leading to toxic effects if not routinely and appropriately monitored.

Cardiovascular Therapies

Antiplatelet Agents

Patients surviving out-of-hospital cardiac arrest who have undergone therapeutic hypothermia often result from acute coronary syndromes and necessitate treatment with coronary angiograph and/or percutaneous coronary intervention (PCI) [58]. Standard treatment strategies prior to and following PCI include the initiation of various antiplatelet agents including glycoprotein IIb/IIIa inhibitors, thienopyridines, and aspirin [59]. There has been considerable research attempting to identify whether therapeutic hypothermia itself induces a state of reduced platelet activation, although some disagreement exists [60–65]. A recent investigation using temperatures commonly seen during therapeutic hypothermia (33–34°C) showed that adenosine diphosphate (ADP)-induced platelet aggregation was unaltered and perhaps slightly elevated versus normothermic controls (37°C) [65]. Thus, studies evaluating the anti-aggregatory effects of commonly used antiplatelet agents is paramount.

The effect of three currently available glycoprotein IIb/IIIa inhibitors on platelet aggregation was investigated with blood samples from six healthy patients without significant coronary disease [60]. The samples were cooled to either 32°C, 34°C, or 37°C with platelet aggregation initiated using ADP 20 μmol/L in the presence or absence of either abciximab, eptifibatide, or tirofiban. While hypothermia (32°C) itself inhibited ADP-induced platelet aggregation, use of submaximal tirofiban and eptifibatide doses provided additive effects. Interestingly, platelet aggregation with abciximab was not significantly altered with hypothermia versus normothermia. The authors concluded that hypothermia adds to the antiplatelet effects of tirofiban and eptifibatide and clinical doses of these agents may have to be modified in this clinical situation. Additional studies in clinical settings are needed in this area.

A study by Michelson and colleagues used a human forearm model to evaluate whether aspirin augments the platelet dysfunction seen during hypothermia [62]. They found that whereas hypothermia itself resulted in a marked prolongation of bleeding time, addition of aspirin only added to this effect minimally. Additionally, aspirin did not significantly augment hypothermia-induced platelet dysfunction using various in vitro laboratory markers such as platelet surface expression of P-selectin and thromboxane B_2. Whether a dose-related effect of aspirin on either platelet activity or bleeding potential exists is currently unknown.

Two clinical studies have evaluated whether use of the thienopyridines agent clopidogrel is altered during hypothermia [65, 66]. These investigations are particularly important given the recent controversies surrounding clopidogrel nonresponsiveness [67, 68]. The first study obtained blood samples from eight healthy volunteers following a single dose of clopidogrel 600 mg [65]. Blood samples were obtained before the dose and 24-h following its administration. They showed a significant increase in maximum platelet aggregation after both 5 and 20 μmol/L ADP at 33°C versus 37°C ($p<0.001$) at 24 h suggesting an attenuation of the antiplatelet effect of clopidogrel. Similar results were shown by Bjelland and colleagues in 25 Caucasian patients given a clopidogrel loading dose (300–600 mg) followed by 75 mg/day for 3 days during therapeutic hypothermia (33–34°C) for cardiac arrest [66]. Using a platelet reactivity index (PRI) <0.5 to denote a satisfactory antiplatelet response, zero patients on day 1 (following the loading dose) and five patients on day 3 achieved this endpoint. This means that all 100% (25/25) of patients studied were resistant to the antiplatelet effect of clopidogrel after receiving a loading dose during therapeutic hypothermia and 70% (20/25) of patients were resistant on day 3. Thus, use of clopidogrel following PCI in acute coronary syndrome patients undergoing therapeutic hypothermia may not provide adequate antiplatelet effects. Whether the newer more potent agents, such as prasugrel and ticagrelor, use of higher clopidogrel doses, or combination with other antiplatelet drugs such as aspirin would be effective in this clinical setting is currently unknown.

Beta-Adrenergic Receptor Blockers

Physiologic cardiovascular responses normally mediated by the β-adrenoreceptors are diminished during reduced core body temperature [69]. Thus, use of beta-adrenergic receptor blockers during periods of hypothermia could result in exaggerated bradycardia or hypotension. An early study by McAllister and colleagues showed that the plasma concentrations of propranolol during periods of hypothermia were significantly higher than normothermic controls [70]. They also showed significant reductions in the apparent volume of distribution ($p<0.001$) and total body clearance ($p<0.005$) of propranolol. More recent studies in patients undergoing cardiac surgery with cardiopulmonary bypass have demonstrated similar results with propranolol, although one study showed that atenolol pharmacokinetics were not significantly affected [71, 72]. Although reduced mean arterial pressures were seen, particularly in those receiving propranolol during periods of hypothermia, no episodes of bradycardia requiring postoperative pacemaker support were reported. Therefore, although the pharmacokinetics of some beta-adrenergic receptor antagonists appear to be altered during hypothermia, this may not apply to all agents within the class and likely affects agents dependent on hepatic metabolism to a greater degree and should be monitored more closely.

Nitroglycerin/Nitroprusside

Comparatively fewer investigations have been conducted on the use of nitroglycerin or nitroprusside during hypothermia. Booth and colleagues studied nitroglycerin administration in 12 patients scheduled for elective coronary artery bypass grafting surgery [73]. A continuous infusion of nitroglycerin was begun during pre-bypass, increased during bypass, and decreased following surgery. Significant decreases in nitroglycerin clearance were seen during hypothermic cardiopulmonary bypass versus normothermic controls ($p<0.05$). It was suggested that the reduced body temperature during surgery decreased the biotransformation of nitroglycerin into its active metabolites including nitric oxide. Thus, nitroglycerin may lose its clinical effectiveness during therapeutic hypothermia.

Sodium nitroprusside is a short-acting vasodilator given as a continuous intravenous infusion in patients with elevated blood pressures. It is metabolized by a nonenzymatic reaction with hemoglobin resulting in release of free cyanide, which is then converted to thiocyanate in the liver and kidney [74, 75]. These metabolites, if accumulated in appreciable amounts, can result in toxicity and death in some circumstances, particularly individuals with reduced renal function. A small investigation of six patients undergoing hypothermic cardiopulmonary bypass studied the metabolism of sodium nitroprusside given as a continuous intravenous infusion [76]. A significant increase in red blood cell cyanide concentrations was seen during hypothermia that lasted until patients were re-warmed. Hypothermia did not affect the release of cyanide from sodium nitroprusside, while the detoxification of cyanide to thiocyanate was delayed until after rewarming. It was hypothesized that the reduced metabolic rates of patients during hypothermia prevented expression of cyanide toxicity while, on rewarming, the detoxification of cyanide kicked in. In summary, it seems as though nitroprusside could be used in patients undergoing therapeutic hypothermia if the clinical situation called for it.

Antimicrobial Agents

Given the prevalence with which antimicrobial agents are given to patients in intensive care units, there is comparatively few data on the affects of hypothermia on this group of pharmacologic agents. Early observations suggested that reducing core body temperature to 19°C for 24 h increased survival in a pneumococcal peritonitis mouse model [77]. An extreme hypothermia (2–4°C) mouse staphylococcal septicemia model showed that penicillin was ineffective at treating the infection, although the relevance of this older study to today's practice can be questioned [78]. More recent data from patients undergoing cardiac surgery with cardiopulmonary bypass showed that vancomycin serum levels are significantly increased during bypass (hypothermia) and normalize during rewarming [79]. This means that patients receiving therapeutic hypothermia following cardiac arrest who require treatment with vancomycin should have their serum drug concentrations followed very closely both during cooling as well as rewarming.

The aminoglycoside antibiotics are the most studies class of antimicrobial agents in various models of hypothermia [80–82]. A piglet model by Koren and colleagues showed that the elimination half-life of gentamicin was significantly prolonged during hypothermia (29°C) versus normothermia (37°C) in addition to decreases in volume of distribution and total body clearance [80]. They authors attributed these changes in pharmacokinetic parameters to decreases in cardiac output and glomerular filtration rate during hypothermia. Similar findings were seen in a small pharmacokinetic case series of neurocritical care patients using the aminoglycoside antibiotic tobramycin where each patient had a slower elimination rate constant and volume of distribution during hypothermia [81]. Interestingly, infant patients with moderate or severe hypoxic-ischemic encephalopathy undergoing hypothermia with core temperatures of 33.5°C saw similar trough serum gentamicin levels versus those kept at normal temperatures [82]. Thus, it appears that different patient populations react to aminoglycoside antibiotics differently and should have serum drug concentrations monitored routinely when therapy is initiated.

Conclusions

Numerous clinical studies show that drug metabolism and elimination is adversely affected during use of therapeutic hypothermia. Drugs such as anesthetics, analgesics, and neuromuscular blockers, which are all used frequently following cardiac arrest, may be affected by lower core body temperatures. One of the challenges facing medical professionals now is how to apply this information to their clinical practice settings. Unfortunately, studies providing more concrete recommendations on handling dosing and monitoring of these medications are lacking and are sorely needed. Until that time, patients should have very close monitoring for both efficacy and well as safety of any pharmacologic agents used during the cooling, maintenance, and rewarming stages of therapeutic hypothermia following cardiac arrest.

References

1. Hachimi-Idrissi S, Corne L, Ebinger G, et al. Mild hypothermia induced by a helmet device: a clinical feasibility study. Resuscitation. 2001;51:275–81.
2. HACA Investigators. Mild therapeutic hypothermia to improve the neurologic outcome after cardiac arrest. N Engl J Med. 2002;346:549–56.
3. Bernard SA, Gray TW, Buist MD, et al. Treatment of comatose survivors of out-of-hospital cardiac arrest with induced hypothermia. N Engl J Med. 2002;346:557–63.
4. Lundbye JB, Rai M, Ramu B, et al. Therapeutic hypothermia is associated with improved neurologic outcomes and survival in cardiac arrest survivors of non-shockable rhythms. Resuscitation. 2012;83:202–7.
5. Polderman KH. Mechamisms of action, physiologic effects, and complications of hypothermia. Crit Care Med. 2009;37(7 Suppl):S186–202.

6. Tortorici MA, Kochanek PM, Poloyac SM. Effects of hypothermia on drug disposition, metabolism, and response: a focus of hypothermia-mediated alterations on the cytochrome P450 enzyme system. Crit Care Med. 2007;35:2196–204.
7. Van den Broek MP, Groenendaal F, Egberts AC, et al. Effects of hypothermia on pharmacokinetics and pharmacodynamics. A systematic review of preclinical and clinical studies. Clin Pharmacokinet. 2010;49:277–94.
8. Zhou J, Poloyac SM. The effect of therapeutic hypothermia on drug metabolism and response: cellular mechanisms to organ function. Expert Opin Drug Metab Toxicol. 2011;7:803–16.
9. Anzenbacher P, Anzenbacherova E. Cytochromes P450 and metabolism of xenobiotics. Cell Mol Life Sci. 2001;58:737–47.
10. Lin JH, Lu AY. Inhibition and induction of cytochrome P450 and the clinical implications. Clin Pharmacokinet. 1998;35:361–90.
11. Fritz HG, Holzmary M, Walter B, et al. The effect of mild hypothermia on plasma fentanyl concentration and biotransformation in juvenile pigs. Anesth Analg. 2005;100:996–1002.
12. Gepts E, Camu F, Cockshott I, et al. Disposition of propofol administered as constant rate intravenous infusions in humans. Anesth Analg. 1987;66:1256–63.
13. Morgan DJ, Campbell GA, Crankshaw DP. Pharmacokinetics of propofol when given by intravenous infusion. Br J Clin Pharmacol. 1990;30:144–8.
14. Cockshott I, Douglas E, Prys-Roberts C, et al. The pharmacokinetics of propofol during and after intravenous infusion in man. Eur J Anaesthesiol. 1990;7:265–75.
15. Jacobi J, Fraser GL, Coursin DB, et al. Clinical practice guidelines for the sustained use of sedatives and analgesics in the critically ill adult. Crit Care Med. 2002;30:119–41.
16. Leslie K, Sessler DI, Bjorksten AR, et al. Mild hypothermia alters propofol pharmacokinetics and increases the duration of action of atracurium. Anesth Analg. 1995;80:1007–14.
17. Kang TM. Propofol infusion syndrome in critically ill patients. Ann Pharmacother. 2002;36:1453–6.
18. Fukuoka N, Aibiki M, Tsukamoto T, et al. Biphasic concentration change during continuous midazolam administration in brain-injured patients undergoing therapeutic moderate hypothermia. Resuscitation. 2004;60:225–30.
19. Hostler D, Zhou J, Tortorici MA. Mild hypothermia alters midazolam pharmacokinetics in normal healthy volunteers. Drug Metab Dispos. 2010;38:781–8.
20. Ariano RE, Kassum DA, Aronson KJ. Comparison of sedative recovery time after midazolam versus diazepam administration. Crit Care Med. 1994;22:1492–6.
21. Malacrida R, Fritz ME, Suter P, et al. Pharmacokinetics of midazolam administered by continuous infusion to intensive care patients. Crit Care Med. 1992;20:1123–6.
22. Bauer TM, Ritz R, Haberthur C, et al. Prolonged sedation due to accumulation of conjugated metabolites of midazolam. Lancet. 1995;246:145–7.
23. Chamorro C, Borrallo JM, Romera MA, et al. Anesthesia and analgesia protocol during therapeutic hypothermia after cardiac arrest: a systematic review. Anesth Analg. 2010;110:1328–35.
24. Holzer M. Targeted temperature management of comatose survivors of cardiac arrest. N Engl J Med. 2010;363:1256–64.
25. Nolan JP, Neumar RW, Adrie C, et al. Post-cardiac arrest syndrome: epidemiology, pathophysiology, treatment, and prognostication. A scientific statement from the International Liaison Committee on Resuscitaiton; the American Heart Association Emergency Cardiovascular Care Committee; the Council on Cardiovascular Surgery and Anesthesia; the Council on Cardiopulmonary, Perioperative, and Critical Care; the Council on Clinical Cardiology; the Council on Stroke. Resuscitation. 2008;19:350–9.
26. Castren M, Silfvast T, Rubertsson S, et al. Scandinavian clinical practice guidelines for therapeutic hypothermia and post-resuscitation care after cardiac arrest. Acta Anaesthesiol Scand. 2009;53:280–8.
27. Murray MJ, Cowen J, DeBlock H, et al. Clinical practice guidelines for sustained neuromuscular blockade in the adult critically ill patient. Crit Care Med. 2002;30:142–56.
28. Warr J, Thiboutot Z, Rose L, et al. Current therapeutic uses, pharmacology, and clinical considerations of neuromuscular blocking agents for critically ill adults. Ann Pharmacother. 2011;45:1116–26.
29. Heier T, Caldwell JE. Impact of hypothermia on the response to neuromuscular blocking drugs. Anesthesiology. 2006;104:1070–80.
30. Miller RD, Agoston S, van der Pol F, et al. Hypothermia and the pharmacokinetics and pharmacodynamics of pancuronium in the cat. J Pharmacol Exp Ther. 1978;207:532–8.
31. Horrow JC, Bartkowski RR. Pancuronium, unlike other nondepolarizing relaxants, retains potency at hypothermia. Anesthesiology. 1983;58:357–61.
32. Beaufort TM, Proost JH, Maring JG, et al. Effect of hypothermia on the hepatic uptake and biliary excretion of vecuronium in the isolated perfused rat liver. Anesthesiology. 2001;94:270–9.
33. Heier T, Caldwell JE, Sessler D, et al. Mild intraoperative hypothermia increases duration of action and spontaneous recovery of vecuronium blockade during nitrous oxide-isoflurane anesthesia in humans. Anesthesiology. 1991;74:815–9.
34. Heier T, Caldwell JE, Sharma ML, et al. Mild intraoperative hypothermia does not change the pharmacodynamics (concentration-effect relationship) of vecuronium in humans. Anesth Analg. 1994;78:973–7.
35. Caldwell JE, Heier T, Wright PMC, et al. Temperature-dependent pharmacokinetics and pharmacodynamics of vecuronium. Anesthesiology. 2000;92:84–93.
36. Cammu G, Coddens J, Hendrickx J, et al. Dose requirements of infusions of Cisatracurium or

rocuronium during hypothermic cardiopulmonary bypass. Br J Anaesth. 2000;84:897–90.
37. Denny NM, Kneeshaw JD. Vecuronium and atracurium infusions during hypothermic cardiopulmonary bypass. Anaesthesia. 1986;41:919–22.
38. Buzello W, Schluermann D, Schindler M, et al. Hypothermic cardiopulmonary bypass and neuromuscular blockade by pancuronium and vecuronium. Anesthesiology. 1985;62:201–4.
39. Diefenbach C, Abel M, Buzello W. Greater neuromuscular blocking potency of atracurium during hypothermic than during normothermic cardiopulmonary bypass. Anesth Analg. 1992;75:275–8.
40. Futter EM, Whalley DG, Wunands JE, et al. Pancuronium requirements during hypothermic cardiopulmonary bypass in man. Anaesth Intensive Care. 1983;11:216–9.
41. Smeulers NJ, Wierda MKJ, van den Boek L, et al. Effects of hypothermic cardiopulmonary bypass on the pharmacodynamics and pharmacokinetics of rocuronium. J Cardiothorac Vasc Anesth. 1995;9: 700–5.
42. McClain DA, Hugg CC. Intravenous fentanyl kinetics. Clin Pharmacol Ther. 1980;28:106–14.
43. Koren G, Barker C, Goresky G, et al. The influence of hypothermia on the disposition of fentanyl – human and animal studies. Eur J Clin Pharmacol. 1987;32: 373–6.
44. Statler KD, Alexander HL, Vagni VA, et al. Moderate hypothermia may be detrimental after traumatic brain injury in fentanyl-anesthetized rats. Crit Care Med. 2003;31:1134–9.
45. Fritz HG, Holzmayr M, Walter B, et al. The effect of mild hypothermia on plasma fentanyl concentration and biotransformation in juvenile pigs. Anesth Analg. 2005;100:996–1002.
46. Empey PE, Miller TM, Philbrick AH, et al. Mild hypothermia decreases fentanyl and midazolam steady-state clearance in a rat model of cardiac arrest. Crit Care Med. 2012;40:1221–8.
47. Koska AJ, Romagnoli A, Kramer WG. Effect of cardiopulmonary bypass on fentanyl distribution and elimination. J Pharmacol Ther. 1981;29:100–5.
48. Koska AJ, Romagnoli A, Kramer WG. Pharmacodynamics of fentanyl citrate in patients undergoing aortocoronary bypass. Cardiovasc Dis. 1981;8: 405–12.
49. Gruber EM, Laussen PC, Costa A, et al. Stress response in infants undergoing cardiac surgery: a randomized study of fentanyl bolus, fentanyl infusion, and fentanyl-midazolam infusion. Anesth Analg. 2001;92:882–90.
50. Kussman BD, Zurakowski D, Sullivan L, et al. Evaluation of plasma fentanyl concentrations in infants during cardiopulmonary bypass with low-volume circuits. J Cardiothorac Vasc Anesth. 2005;19: 316–21.
51. Ruggeri L, Landoni G, Guarracino F, et al. Remifentanil in critically ill cardiac patients. Ann Card Anaesth. 2011;14:6–12.
52. Burkle H, Dunbar S, Van Aken H. Remifentanil: a novel, short-acting, mu-opioid. Anesth Analg. 1996; 83:646–51.
53. Russell D, Royston D, Rees PH, et al. Effect of temperature and cardiopulmonary bypass on the pharmacokinetics of remifentanil. Br J Anaesth. 1997;79:456–9.
54. Michelsen LG, Golford NHG, Lu W, et al. The pharmacokinetics of remifentanil in patients undergoing coronary artery bypass grafting with cardiopulmonary bypass. Anesth Analg. 2001;93:1100–5.
55. Puig MM, Warner W, Tang CK, et al. Effects of temperature on the interaction of morphine with opioid receptors. Br J Anaesth. 1987;59:1459–64.
56. Bansinath M, Turndorf H, Puig MM. Influence of hypo and hyperthermia on disposition of morphine. J Clin Pharmacol. 1988;28:860–4.
57. Roka A, Melinda KT, Vasarhelyi B, et al. Elevated morphine concentrations in neonates treated with morphine and prolonged hypothermia for hypoxic ischemic encephalopathy. Pediatrics. 2008;121:e844–9.
58. Nielsen N, Hovdenes J, Nilsson F, et al. Outcome, timing, and adverse events in therapeutic hypothermia after out-of-hospital cardiac arrest. Acta Anaesthesiol Scand. 2009;53:926–34.
59. Harrington RA, Becker RC, Cannon CP, et al. Antithrombotic therapy for non-ST-segment elevation acute coronary syndromes: American College of Chest Physicians evidence-based clinical practice guidelines (8th edition). Chest. 2008;133(6 Suppl):670S–707.
60. Frelinger AL, Furman MI, Barnard MR, et al. Combined effects of mild hypothermia and glycoprotein IIb/IIIa antagonists on platelet-platelet and leukocyte-platelet aggregation. Am J Cardiol. 2003;92: 1099–101.
61. Michelson AD, MacGregor H, Barnard MR, et al. Reversible inhibition of human platelet activation by hypothermia in vivo and in vitro. Thromb Haemost. 1994;71:633–40.
62. Michelson AD, Barnard MR, Khuri SF, et al. The effects of aspirin and hypothermia on platelet function in vivo. Br J Haematol. 1999;104:64–8.
63. Lindenblatt N, Menger MD, Klar E, et al. Sustained hypothermia accelerates microvascular thrombus formation in mice. Am J Physiol Heart Circ Physiol. 2005;289:H2680–7.
64. Xavier G, Kalb M, Marschalek C, et al. The effects of test temperature and storage temperature on platelet aggregation: a whole blood in vitro study. Anesth Analg. 2006;102:1280–4.
65. Hogberg C, Erlinge D, Braun OO. Mild hypothermia does not attenuate platelet aggregation and may even increase ADP-stimulated platelet aggregation after clopidogrel treatment. Thromb J. 2009;7:2.
66. Bjelland TW, Hjertner O, Klepstad P, et al. Antiplatelet effect of clopidogrel is reduced in patients treated with therapeutic hypothermia after cardiac arrest. Resuscitation. 2010;81:1627–31.
67. Nguyen TA, Diodati JG, Pharand C. Resistance to clopidogrel: a review of the evidence. J Am Coll Cardiol. 2001;45:1157–64.

68. O'Donoghue M, Wiviott SD. Clopidogrel response variability and future therapies: clopidogrel: does on size fit all? Circulation. 2006;114:e600–6.
69. Han YS, Tveita T, Kondratiev TV, et al. Changes in cardiovascular β-adrenoceptor responses during hypothermia. Cryobiology. 2008;57:246–50.
70. McAllister RG, Bourne DW, Tan TG, et al. Effects of hypothermia on propranolol kinetics. Clin Pharmacol Ther. 1979;25:1–7.
71. Carmona MJC, Malbouisson LMS, Pereira VA, et al. Cardiopulmonary bypass alters the pharmacokinetics of propranolol in patients undergoing cardiac surgery. Braz J Med Biol Res. 2005;38:713–21.
72. Carmona MJC, Pereira VA, Malbouisson LMS, et al. Effect of cardiopulmonary bypass on the pharmacokinetics of propranolol and atenolol. Braz J Med Biol Res. 2009;42:574–81.
73. Booth BP, Brien JF, Marks GS, et al. The effects of hypothermic and normothermic cardiopulmonary bypass on glyceryl trinitrate activity. Anesth Analg. 1994;78:848–56.
74. Smith RP, Kruszyana H. Nitroprusside produces cyanide poisoning via a reaction with hemoglobin. J Pharmacol Exp Ther. 1974;191:557–63.
75. Tinker JH, Michenfelder JD. Sodium nitroprusside: pharmacology, toxicology, and therapeutics. Anesthesiology. 1976;45:349–54.
76. Moore RA, Guller EA, Gallagher JD, et al. Effect of hypothermic cardiopulmonary bypass on nitroprusside metabolism. Clin Pharmacol Ther. 1985; 37:680–3.
77. Wotkyns RS, Hirose H, Eiseman B. Prolonged hypothermia in experimental pneumococcal peritonitis. Surg Gynecol Obstet. 1958;107:363–9.
78. Jones JH, Campbell PJ. Penicillin therapy of experimental staphylococcal septicemia in mice exposed to cold. J Pathol Bacteriol. 1962;84:433–7.
79. Klamerus KJ, Rodvold KA, Silverman NA, et al. Effect of cardiopulmonary bypass on vancomycin and netilmicin disposition. Antimicrob Agents Chemother. 1988;32:631–5.
80. Koren G, Barker C, Bohn D, et al. Influence of hypothermia on the pharmacokinetics of gentamicin and theophylline in piglets. Crit Care Med. 1985;13: 844–7.
81. Mercer JM, Neyens RR. Aminoglycoside pharmacokinetic parameters in neurocritical care patients undergoing induced hypothermia. Pharmacotherapy. 2010;30:654–60.
82. Liu X, Borooah M, Stone J, et al. Serum gentamicin concentrations in encephalopathic infants are not affected by therapeutic hypothermia. Pediatrics. 2009; 124:310–5.

Determination of Neurological Prognosis

10

Cara Klajbor and Erica Schuyler

After a patient undergoes therapeutic hypothermia (TH) and rewarming is achieved, a neurologist is often involved to prognosticate, especially in difficult cases when the patient remains in a coma. The neurologist must use both the clinical exam and various other data including electrophysiological tests to make a conclusion and suggest the most likely outcome for the patient to the primary team and family. This chapter will review the most current evidence from literature regarding the various elements used to make a prognosis.

Measuring Outcome

The most commonly used scale to report outcomes for patients after cardiac-arrest is the Glasgow-Pittsburgh Cerebral Performance Categories (CPC) [1, 2] (Fig. 10.1). A CPC of 3–5 represents a poor outcome while a CPC of 1–2 represents a good outcome.

C. Klajbor, M.D.
Department of Neurology, Hartford Hospital, 80 Seymour Street, Hartford 06514, CT, USA
e-mail: cklajbor@resident.uchc.edu

E. Schuyler, M.D. (✉)
Department of Neurology, Hartford Hospital/University of Connecticut, Hartford CT, USA

Department of Medicine, University of Connecticut School of Medicine, Farmington, CT, USA
e-mail: eschuyler@harthosp.org

History and Current Guidelines

Because TH has only recently become more widely used, much of the scientific literature currently available addresses prognosis after cardiac arrest without taking into account the added variable of hypothermia. One of the fundamental studies that established a model for prognostication was published by Levy et al. in 1985. This study found that in patients with cerebral hypoxia-ischemia, the factors that were most useful in prognosticating a poor outcome were absent pupillary reflexes at initial exam, and at 24 h, absent, flexor or extensor motor responses and spontaneous eye movements that were neither orientating or roving conjugate [3].

Since this study, a comprehensive set of guidelines was published in 2006 for prognostication after cardiac arrest. These most current practice parameters from the American Academy of Neurology (AAN) were created through analyzing studies performed from 1966 to 2006 [4]. The guidelines expanded the list of variables from those in the Levy et al. study and took into account circumstances surrounding CPR, increased body temperature, neurological exam, electrophysiological tests, biochemical markers, neuroimaging and monitoring of intracranial pressure and brain oxygenation. It was found that elevated body temperature, intracranial pressure, brain oxygenation, and the circumstances surrounding CPR, such as time length of CPR, cause of arrest, and time between arrest and start of CPR cannot be used for prognostication. In the following pages,

J.B. Lundbye (ed.), *Therapeutic Hypothermia After Cardiac Arrest*,
DOI 10.1007/978-1-4471-2951-6_10, © Springer-Verlag London 2012

Fig. 10.1 The Glasgow-Pittsburgh Cerebral Performance Categories (CPC) [1, 2]

CPC 1	Recovery with return to full function of activities of daily living. May have mild cognitive or neurological deficits on exam.
CPC 2	Moderately disabled but independent with activties of daily living. Able to be employed.
CPC 3	Severe neurologic disability and dependent for activities of daily living.
CPC 4	Coma or vegetative state.
CPC 5	Brain death or death.

the results of analysis of the other variables in the guidelines are set forth by category along with evidence from recent studies examining the way hypothermia may effect these recommendations. Prognostication after the advent of hypothermia is challenging, and the timing of the neurological assessment and thus decisions to withdraw care may be altered [5].

Neurological Examination

The AAN guidelines state that absence of pupillary or corneal reflexes within 1–3 days, or absent or extensor responses 3 days after cardiac arrest accurately predict poor outcome [4]. The optimal timing of the neurological exam has yet to be identified in TH patients due to limited data and current studies have sought to test whether these guidelines remain accurate in TH patients.

Performing a neurological exam for prognosis during hypothermia and before rewarming is not recommended as the accuracy of the findings can be altered by the effect of hypothermia on the normal physiology of organ systems. Drug clearance, specifically for paralytic agents, opiates and sedatives, is reduced when body temperature drops below 35°C [6]. Also, these medications are used more frequently in hypothermia patients within 12 h of the 72 h neurological exam [7]. Despite the effects of sedation, one recent study of 227 prospectively identified cardiac-arrest survivors did not identify a difference in time to regaining consciousness when comparing TH and non-TH patients, reporting that the median time in both groups was 2 days after cardiac arrest with the majority awakening within 3 days [8]. This study did have patients in both groups that regained consciousness after the fifth day. However, confounding variables such as severe systemic illness and differing rates of sedative drug metabolism may have contributed to this.

A withdrawal response on motor exam within 24 h of weaning sedation has been found to be indicative of good prognosis [9]. On the other hand, some studies have found that poor response on the motor component of the exam is less reliable for poor prognosis prediction in hypothermia patients [7, 10]. In a retrospective chart review of 37 patients, 2 of 14 patients who showed a motor response no better than extension on day 3 later regained awareness, but did not show good motor response until 6 days after arrest [10]. At 72 h after cardiac arrest, absent pupillary and corneal responses, and myoclonic status epilepticus remained highly predictive of poor outcome in this study. A prospective study of 85 post-CPR comatose patients examining the effects of sedation on different elements of the neurological assessment found that both poor motor response and absence of corneal reflexes are not accurate at 72 h in patients who received sedation within 12 h of the exam regardless of whether they underwent TH, while absent pupillary response and myoclonic status epilepticus still could accurately predict poor prognosis [7]. Another prospective study of 111 TH patients found higher false positive rates for absence of pupillary reactivity and corneal reflexes, myoclonic status epilepticus, and motor response at 72 h in TH patients compared to those reported in the AAN guidelines [11]. Given these variable findings, the neurological exam should be used with caution for prognostication in TH patients. Evidence suggests that a poor motor response is not as reliable in hypothermia patients most likely due to sedation, while a good motor response predicts favorable outcome. Lack of pupillary reactivity and corneal reflexes at 72 h suggests a poor prognosis but not with absolute certainty, so the use of other modalities in conjunction with the exam is suggested.

Neuroimaging

According to the guideline recommendations, there is inadequate data to support whether neuroimaging features such as diffuse swelling on computed tomography (CT) of the head or signal changes on magnetic resonance imaging (MRI) of the brain can be used to predict poor outcome [4]. MRI diffusion-weighted imaging (DWI) with apparent diffusion coefficient (ADC) is commonly used after cardiac arrest and can allow visualization of the degree of anoxic brain injury and ischemia. Recent studies on hypothermia patients have shown that in the patients that have a poor outcome, the diffusion lesions are both more numerous and larger than in patients that survive [12, 13]. Another study has found that when DWI is performed within 5 days of cardiac arrest, the location of the injury is also important, and a mixed pattern of injury involving the cortex and deep grey nuclei may correlate with a poor outcome [14]. Overall, there is no evidence to support that imaging can be used in isolation to predict clinical outcome. DWI can show changes 3–5 days after CA and as early as 3 days after cardiac arrest, diffuse brain swelling can be seen on non-contrast head CT.

Somatosensory Evoked Potentials

The AAN guidelines report that bilateral absence of the N20 component of somatosensory evoked potentials (SSEPs) with median nerve stimulation 1–3 days post cardiac arrest accurately predicts poor outcome [4]. The cortical N20 refers to a negative peak (N) at 20 ms and is recorded from the cortex when the median nerve is stimulated. These responses are known to be affected by temperature and hypothermia can alter the amplitude and prolong the latency of the evoked potentials [14]. In a prospective, randomized, controlled trial of 60 cardiac arrest patients randomized to either hypothermia or normothermia groups, the results of SSEPs performed at 24–28 h after cardiac arrest showed that even though wave latencies are significantly prolonged in the hypothermia patients, absence of bilateral N20 responses in TH patients is still an accurate predictor of poor outcome [15]. However, one retrospective study of 36 TH patients with absence of bilateral N20 response at 72 h showed that one patient did regain consciousness and have a good outcome [16]. SSEPs can be a difficult test to perform in the ICU and many institutions may have limited access to this resource. While absence of the N20 response remains an indicator of poor prognosis in hypothermia patients, it cannot be used alone to predict with complete accuracy.

Electroencephalogram (EEG)

EEG has long been studied for its effectiveness in prognostication in CA patients. AAN guidelines suggest that generalized suppression to ≤20 μV, burst-suppression pattern with generalized epileptiform activity, or generalized periodic complexes on a flat background are strongly but not invariably associated with poor outcome [4]. Recent AHA guidelines recommend a routine EEG 24 h or more after cardiac arrest for patients not treated with hypothermia protocol, although there is no definite recommendation for TH patients [17]. Recent studies have found that during hypothermia, unreactive EEG was highly indicative of mortality, and an initial flat background on amplitude integrated EEG had no prognostic value [18, 19]. These studies as well as studies performed after return of normothermia have been consistent with the AAN guidelines, finding that discontinuous burst-suppression or generalized epileptiform activity was indicative of poor prognosis [20]. Based on available evidence, a burst-suppression pattern and lack of reactivity on EEG indicate poor prognosis. EEG, either routine length or continuous video-EEG monitoring, can be useful during hypothermia in order to detect seizures that may be non-convulsive or have motor manifestations masked by paralytic drugs so that treatment may be initiated [21]. After return of normothermia, the EEG background activity can be used in addition to other criteria to make a prognosis.

Status Epilepticus

According to the AAN guidelines, prognosis is poor in comatose patients diagnosed with myoclonic status epilepticus within 1 day of primary circulatory arrest [4]. Postanoxic status epilepticus (PSE) is often found in patients after CA and has been shown to be associated with mortality [22]. However, one study of six TH patients that regained consciousness despite PSE (3 myoclonic and 3 non-convulsive) treated with anti-epileptic medications showed that these patients all had preserved brainstem reflexes, present SSEPs, and EEG reactivity [23]. Other studies in TH patients have substantiated the finding that myoclonic status epilepticus after hypothermia is indicative of poor prognosis [7, 10]. Paralytic agents used during hypothermia may delay diagnosis of myoclonic status epilepticus, and detecting it clinically in the first 24 h, as mentioned in the guidelines, may not be possible without an EEG. PSE, including myoclonic status epilepticus, may not invariably predict poor outcome especially in patients with other favorable characteristics and more studies need to be performed to assess the usefulness of aggressive treatment of PSE.

Biomarkers

AAN guidelines state that a Neuron-specific enolase (NSE) level >33 μg/L at days 1–3 post-cardiac arrest accurately predicts poor outcome [4]. NSE is a biochemical marker that can be measured in both the serum and CSF and is released by neurons during injury such as in the setting of hypoxia, as well as by erythrocytes and platelets [24]. The current literature regarding NSE shows varying results regarding the cut-off value for zero false positives for predicting poor outcome in hypothermia patients [25]. While some studies have substantiated the NSE cut-off value of >33 μg/L, others have shown that increases in NSE when measured in TH patients over days may indicate poor prognosis [24, 26]. The variability in the cut-off values, most likely due to lack of standardization of variables such as time of sampling, makes NSE an unreliable predictor at this time.

Conclusion

Although there are no current guidelines about making a prognosis in patients treated with hypothermia, we must deduce information from emerging literature and guidelines available pre-hypothermia. A timeline of the various modalities used for diagnosis based on current studies is summarized in Fig. 10.2.

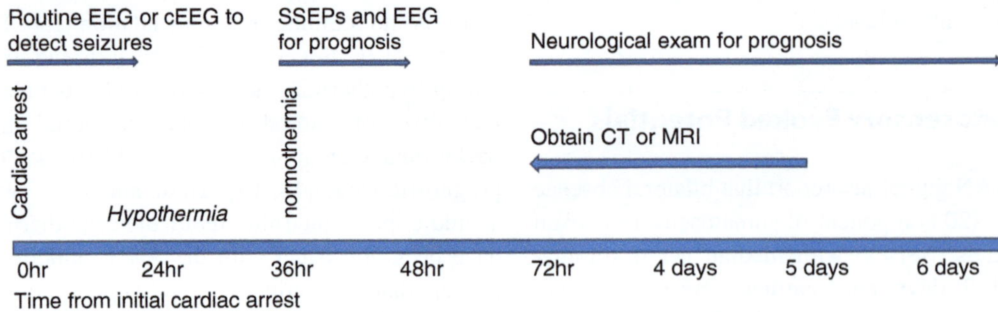

Fig. 10.2 Timeline to obtain elements of the neurological assessment in therapeutic hypothermia patients

An important aspect to keep in mind is that the results of outcome studies may be biased by the self-fulfilling prophecy in which those patients that are considered to have a poor prognosis and undergo withdrawal of care may not survive long enough to exhibit improved neurological status. This is why it is important for physicians involved in the care of these patients to be conscientious about when the neurological exam and other tests are performed and when it is appropriate to conclude that prognosis for neurological recovery is dismal. The best approach to determining prognosis is one in which several modalities are used, as no single finding is completely reliable in those patients undergoing therapeutic hypothermia.

References

1. Jennett B, Bond M. Assessment of outcome after severe brain damage. Lancet. 1975;305:480–4.
2. Cummings RO, Chamberlain DA, Abramson NS, et al. Recommended guidelines for uniform reporting of data from out-of-hospital cardiac arrest: the Utstein style. Circulation. 1991;84:960–75.
3. Levy DE, Caronna JJ, Singer BH, et al. Predicting outcome from hypoxic-ischemic coma. JAMA. 1985;253: 1420–6.
4. Wiijdicks EFM, Hijdra A, Young BG, Report of the Quality Standards Subcommittee of the American Academy of Neurology, et al. Practice parameter: prediction of outcome in comatose survivors after cardiopulmonary resuscitation (an evidence-based review). Neurology. 2006;67:203–10.
5. Perman SM, Kirkpatrick JN, Reitsma AM, et al. Timing of neuroprognostication in postcardiac arrest therapeutic protocol. Crit Care Med. 2012;40:1–6.
6. Polderman KH. Application of therapeutic hypothermia in the intensive care unit. Opportunities and pitfalls of a promising treatment modality. Part 2: practical aspects and side effects. Intensive Care Med. 2004;30:757–69.
7. Samiengo EA, Mlynash M, Caulfield AF, et al. Sedation confounds outcome prediction in cardiac arrest survivors treated with hypothermia. Neurocrit Care. 2010;15:113–9.
8. Fugate JE, Wijdicks EFM, White RD, et al. Does therapeuric hypothermia affect time to awakening in cardiac arrest survivors? Neurology. 2011;77: 1346–50.
9. Schefold JC, Storm C, Kruger A, et al. The Glasgow Coma Score is a predictor of good outcome in cardiac arrest patients treated with therapeutic hypothermia. Resuscitation. 2009;80:658–61.
10. Al Thenayan E, Savard M, Sharpe M, et al. Predictors of poor neurologic outcome after induced mild hypothermia following cardiac arrest. Neurology. 2008;71:1535–7.
11. Rossetti A, Oddo M, Logroscino G. Prognostication after cardiac arrest and hypothermia; a prospective study. Ann Neurol. 2010;67:301–7.
12. Jarnum H, Knutsson L, Rundgren M, et al. Diffusion and perfusion MRI of the brain in comatose patients treated with mild hypothermia after cardiac arrest: a prospective observational study. Resuscitation. 2009;80:425–30.
13. Wijdicks EF, Campeau NG, Miller GM. MR imaging in comatose survivors of cardiac resuscitation. AJNR Am J Neuroradiol. 2001;22:1561–5.
14. Lang M, Welte M, Hansen D. Effects of hypothermia on median nerve somatosensory evoked potential during spontaneous circulation. J Neurosurg Anesthesiol. 2002;14:141–5.
15. Tiainen M, Kovala T, Takkunen O, et al. Somatosensory and brainstem auditory evoked potentials in cardiac arrest patients treated with hypothermia. Crit Care Med. 2005;33:1736–40.
16. Leithner C, Pioner CJ, Hasper D, et al. Does hypothermia influence the predictive value of bilateral absent N20 after cardiac arrest. Neurology. 2010; 74:965–9.
17. Peberdy MA, Callaway CW, Neumar RW, et al. Post-cardiac arrest care: 2010 American Heart Association Guidelines for cardiopulmonary resuscitation and emergency cardiovascular care. Circulation. 2010;122: S768–86.
18. Rossetti AO, Urbano LA, Delodder F, et al. Prognostic value of continuous EEG monitoring during therapeutic hypothermia protocol after cardiac arrest. Crit Care. 2010;14:R173.
19. Rundgren M, Westhall E, Cronberg T, et al. Continuous amplitude-integrated electroencephalogram predicts outcome in hypothermia-treated cardiac arrest patients. Crit Care Med. 2010;38: 1838–44.
20. Al Thenayan E, Savard M, Sharpe M, et al. Electroencephalogram for prognosis after cardiac arrest. J Crit Care. 2010;25:300–4.
21. Hovland A, Nielson EW, Kluver J, et al. EEG should be performed during induced hypothermia. Resuscitation. 2006;68:143–6.
22. Rossetti A, Logrscino G, Liaudet L, et al. Status epilepticus: an independent outcome predictor after cerebral anoxia. Neurology. 2007;69:255–60.
23. Rossetti A, Oddo M, Liaudet L, et al. Predictors of awakening from postanoxic status epilepticus after therapeutic hypothermia. Neurology. 2009;72: 744–9.
24. Rundgren M, Karlsson T, Nielson N, et al. Neuron specific enolase and S-100B as predictors of outcome

after cardiac arrest and induced hypothermia. Resuscitation. 2009;80:784–9.

25. Daubin C, Quentin C, Allouche A, et al. Serum-specific enolase as predictor of outcome in comatose cardiac-arrest survivors: a prospective cohort study. BMC Cardiovasc Disord. 2011;11:1–13.

26. Oksanen T, Tiainen M, Skrifvars M, et al. Predictive power of serum NSE and OHCA score regarding 6-month neurologic outcome aft out-of-hospital ventricular fibrillation and therapeutic hypothermia. Resuscitation. 2009;80:165–70.

11 Therapeutic Hypothermia as a Treatment of Myocardial Infarction and Cardiogenic Shock

David Erlinge

Introduction

Mild hypothermia (32–35°C) has been shown to reduce mortality and improve neurological outcome in unconscious patients suffering cardiac arrest [1, 2], and is recommended by treatment guidelines [3]. This raises the question of whether it is possible to use hypothermia to limit or prevent the damage caused to the heart during ST-elevation myocardial infarction (STEMI).

Hypothermia is a well established method of protecting the heart during coronary artery bypass grafting [4]. It is also crucial for successful heart transplantation as it protects the donor heart after explantation. However, in these circumstances deep hypothermia (<30°C) is often used, which may cause spontaneous ventricular fibrillation, leading to the need for circulatory support. Thus, in order to treat conscious patients with STEMI, cardiologists are restricted in using hypothermia within the range 32–35°C(mild). Interestingly, even mild hypothermia has the ability to protect the heart against the development of myocardial infarction. In a large number of animal studies, the protective effect has been found to range from 18% to 90% when hypothermia was started during ischemia, in the rat, rabbit, dog and pig [5, 6]. Furthermore, small clinical safety and feasibility studies have shown promising effects [7].

D. Erlinge, M.D., Ph.D.
Department of Cardiology, Lund University,
Skane University Hospital, Lund SE-221 85, Sweden
e-mail: david.erlinge@med.lu.se

Cardioprotection: The Next Treatment Opportunity

The current treatment of acute STEMI is to open the occluded coronary artery and to reperfuse the ischemic myocardium using either thrombolysis or primary percutaneous coronary intervention (PCI) as soon as possible, in order to reduce the extent of the infarction and associated complications. Infarct size is one of the main predictors of both short- and long-term outcome in patients with acute myocardial infarction (AMI) [8, 9]. Additional antithrombotic therapy can be used to help keep the artery open. Paradoxically, the actual process of restoring coronary blood flow to previously ischemic myocardium can in itself increase the myocardial injury sustained during ischemia—a phenomenon termed myocardial reperfusion injury [10–12]. Reperfusion injury causes four types of cardiac dysfunction: (1) myocardial stunning, (2) microvascular obstruction or no-reflow phenomenon, (3) reperfusion arrhythmia, and (4) lethal reperfusion injury [13]. Lethal reperfusion injury is defined as cardiomyocyte death mediated by reperfusion and not by the ischemia alone. Hypothermia may have beneficial effects on all these kinds of reperfusion injuries, but the focus of this review is on lethal reperfusion injury.

J.B. Lundbye (ed.), *Therapeutic Hypothermia After Cardiac Arrest*,
DOI 10.1007/978-1-4471-2951-6_11,

Promising or Failed Cardioprotective Strategies

Previous attempts to limit this form of myocardial injury in patients after STEMI using pharmacological strategies as adjuncts to primary PCI have often worked well in animal studies, and appeared promising in small clinical phase I or II studies, but have generally failed in larger randomized clinical trials [14–16]. Several mechanisms are involved in reperfusion injury [13]. The problem with previous cardioprotective agents could be that they only affect one single mechanism per treatment. Hypothermia has the advantage of affecting a wide range of mechanisms, and this may be important in achieving clinical effects.

Early Animal Experiments Using Mild Hypothermia for Acute Myocardial Infarction

It has been known for over 30 years that deep hypothermia (<30°C) reduces the extent of myocardial infarction [17]. However, the detrimental physiological effect of deep hypothermia on the heart (spontaneous ventricular fibrillation and reduced ventricular function) makes it less suitable for treating conscious patients. The first study to demonstrate cardioprotective effects of mild hypothermia in myocardial ischemia found a linear correlation between infarct size, in relation to the area at risk, and temperature in the interval from 35°C to 42°C in rabbits subjected to 30 min coronary occlusion; the size of the infarct being decreased by 8% for each degree of temperature reduction [18]. At a temperature of 35°C complete protection was achieved and no infarction was seen. Although pre-ischemia cooling studies are important in demonstrating the powerful cardioprotective effects of hypothermia, the protocol cannot be applied to humans, as patients do not present at the hospital before STEMI occurs. It is important to note that not only does lowering the body temperature below 37°C reduce infarct size; but that elevated temperature increases infarct size, indicating that fever should be treated in patients with acute myocardial infarction [18–20].

Application of hypothermia after the onset of ischemia could substantially reduce infarct size, and that the longer the period of hypothermia during ischemia, the better the cardioprotective effect [21–23]. In a review by Tissier and coworkers, the results of 16 studies on the effect of hypothermia during ischemia are summarized in a structured table. A reduction in myocardial infarct size was found in all these studies, ranging from 18% to 90% [5]. These results are important as they demonstrate that inducing hypothermia after the onset of ischemia reduces damage to the heart, and thus that clinically applicable protocols in this regard can be developed.

Another aspect of reperfusion injury, myocardial stunning, is also prevented by hypothermia. This has been shown in a rabbit model in which myocardial function measured as segment length shortening, was significantly increased in the hypothermia-treated animals [24].

A multitude of cooling methods have been used in animal experiments: topical cooling using ice in the open chest [22], cold perfusion of the pericardium [25], intracoronary infusions [26], hypothermic coronary retroperfusion [27] and extracorporeal circuit cooling [28], but most of them are too complex or too dangerous to be used in a conscious patient with myocardial infarction.

A pivotal animal study in the development of hypothermia treatment in the clinical setting was carried out by Dae et al. [29]. They used an endovascular heat-exchange cooling catheter designed for clinical use, inserted into the vena cava via the femoral vein, in human-sized pigs subjected to a 60-min occlusion of the left anterior descending artery [29]. Cooling was initiated after 20 min of ischemia, and resulted in an 80% reduction in the size of the infarct in relation to the area at risk [29]. The transferability of the protocol and the impressive effect led to the initiation of two large clinical trials, the COOL-MI and the ICE-IT trials.

Early Clinical Trials of Hypothermia for STEMI

Small clinical trials have demonstrated the safety and feasibility of cooling conscious patients with acute myocardial infarction [30, 31]. Dixon et al.

randomized 42 patients to endovascular heat-exchange cooling or standard PCI treatment [30]. Cooling was well tolerated, with no hemodynamic instability or increase in arrhythmia, and a non-significant trend towards reduction in infarct size was seen. In the LOWTEMP-study, Kandzari et al. treated 18 non-randomized patients with endovascular cooling as adjunctive therapy to primary PCI [31]. Periprocedural endovascular cooling successfully decreased the core body temperature and was well tolerated. In the NICAMI study, surface cooling was tested in cases of acute myocardial infarction [32]. Cooling was well tolerated and safe, but it took 79 min on average to reach the target temperature showing that surface cooling is too slow for STEMI treatment.

Two clinical trials investigating mild hypothermia using endovascular cooling catheters as an adjunct therapy for STEMI, failed to show a reduction in infarct size [14–16]. In the COOL-MI trial (Zoll), 392 STEMI patients were randomized to standard PCI or endovascular cooling for 3 h followed by 4 h re-warming, in addition to PCI. The door-to-balloon time was 18 min longer in the hypothermia group. Nearly all the patients subjected to hypothermia (94%) tolerated the complete cooling protocol well, however, no significant difference was found in the clinical endpoints, serious side effects or in the primary endpoint which was infarct size measured with SPECT after 30 min. In a post-hoc analysis of anterior infarcts in patients who had reached a temperature below 35°C at the onset of reperfusion, a trend towards a 49% reduction in infarct size was seen.

In the ICE-IT trial (Innercool, Philips), 228 STEMI patients were randomized to standard PCI or endovascular cooling for 6 h followed by 3 h re-warming in addition to PCI [15]. No significant differences were found in clinical endpoints or serious side effects. A higher number of deaths were observed in the hypothermia group (9 vs. 4) which could be explained by an excess of elderly patients in the hypothermia group. However, this had effect on the primary endpoint which was infarct size as measured with SPECT after 30 days, as according to the protocol, a patients not surviving was imputed to have the largest infarct size detected. However, when the data were analyzed without imputed values, there was a trend towards a 23% reduction in infarct size in the hypothermia group (PCI: 13.2% vs. PCI+hypothermia: 10.2%, $p=0.14$). In a post-hoc analysis of anterior infarcts in patients who reached a temperature below <35°C at the onset of reperfusion there was a trend towards a 43% reduction in infarct size (PCI: 22.7%, $n=38$ vs. PCI+hypothermia: 12.9%, $n=10$, $p=0.09$).

Interest in hypothermia as a form of treatment for STEMI was considerably reduced after these trials were presented in 2002 and 2003, as the cooling rate was relatively slow, and only a minority of the patients (approximately 30%) had reached a temperature below 35°C at the onset of reperfusion. The post-hoc analysis of the two trials showing strong trends towards a positive effect in patients who did reach a temperature <35°C was highly interesting, but has yet to be verified in animal experiments and prospective clinical trials.

Timing, Speed of Induction and Duration of Hypothermia

Hypothermia during the period of ischemia reduces infarct size. Furthermore, reperfusion injury alone may account for as much as 50% of the final size of the infarct [13]. The post-hoc analysis of the data from the COOL-MI and ICE-IT trials suggests that hypothermia was only effective if a sufficiently low temperature was achieved before reperfusion. In order to induce more rapid cooling we tried to combine endovascular cooling, with a fast infusion of 1 l cold saline in 40–45 kg pigs, and were able to cool the pigs to below 35°C within 5 min [7]. When cooling was instigated immediately after reperfusion, no effect on infarct size was seen, despite reaching a body temperature of 35°C 5 min after reperfusion. This confirmed the post-hoc analysis of the clinical studies regarding the lack of effect of post-reperfusion cooling. When hypothermia was initiated 15 min before reperfusion during a 40 min period of ischemia, the size of the infarct was reduced by 39%. This meant that the pigs had received therapeutic hypothermia for 10 min of the total 40 min period of ischemia, and this could have been responsible for the whole effect.

To ascertain whether hypothermia has an effect on reperfusion injury *per se*, the ischemic period was extended by 5 min and the extra time was used to induce hypothermia [33]. Thus, the two groups had undergone the same period of normothermic ischemia. The size of the infarct was reduced by 18%, proving that hypothermia has a separate effect on reperfusion injury, independent of the effect on ischemia [33]. This 18% reduction is probably an underestimation as the comparison was made with a 5 min shorter period of ischemia. In this way, we confirmed the results of the post-hoc analysis of the data from the COOL-MI and ICE-IT studies that hypothermia is effective before reperfusion and is without effect after reperfusion.

Duration of Hypothermia

The evidence shows that cooling should be achieved as early as possible during ischemia, and should reach as low temperature as possible before reperfusion. However, it is still not known how long after reperfusion cooling should continue. This question also remains unanswered in the case of hypothermia for cardiac arrest. We extended the post-reperfusion cooling in our pig model from 15 to 60 min post-reperfusion, without finding any additional effects on infarct size [33]. This is in agreement with the lack of effect of hypothermia when instigated after the start of reperfusion. This indicates that hypothermia could be terminated quite early after reperfusion. At the same time, it is important that the subject's whole body is thoroughly cooled. Cold saline alone cools the body quickly, but gives a rapid rebound in temperature resulting in a lack of effect on infarct size [33]. We concluded that the 3–6 h post-reperfusion cooling used in the COOL-MI and ICE-IT studies is unnecessarily long and could be shortened to 1 h.

Microvascular Obstruction

Every coronary interventionist performing primary PCI is aware of and often frustrated by, a phenomenon called no-reflow or TIMI 2 flow. Upon opening the occluded epicardial coronary artery a good blood flow is obtained (TIMI 3). However, within a few minutes the flow is restricted by poor run-off in the microcirculation. Histologically, this represents a microvascular obstruction [34]. The mechanism is not fully understood, but involves inflammatory and complement activation, endothelial swelling, red blood cell extravasation and tissue edema. The phenomenon is prevalent in large myocardial infarctions and is correlated with the duration of the myocardial infarction [35].

The presence of microvascular obstruction is independently associated with impaired recovery of left ventricular function and a poor long-term clinical outcome [36, 37]. Hale et al. found that hypothermia reduced microvascular obstruction (measured with microspheres) to a greater extent than infarct size in rabbits [7, 38]. This phenomenon was confirmed in our pig model, where hypothermia reduced the infarct size by 39%, while microvascular obstruction was completely abolished [7]. Furthermore, hypothermia initiated post-reperfusion by cold saline alone reduced microvascular obstruction although it did not result in any reduction in infarct size [7, 33]. These findings indicate that infarct size and microvascular obstruction are, at least partly, separate mechanisms, and link microvascular obstruction to reperfusion injury (Fig. 11.1).

The RAPID MI-ICE Clinical Trial

After seeing the rapid cooling effects of the combination of cold saline and endovascular cooling in our pig model, we investigated whether this combination could increase the number of patients achieving a temperature <35°C before reperfusion. In the COOL-MI and ICE-IT studies only approximately 30% reached <35°C before reperfusion (26% in anterior infarcts in COOL-MI , and 34% in ICE-IT). At the same time, we and other colleagues were concerned that administering a large volume of cold saline, up to 2 L, to patients with large infarctions might cause acute heart failure or pulmonary congestion. We therefore designed the RAPID MI-ICE clinical as a safety and feasibility study on 20 patients with large STEMI treated with primary PCI [39]. The study showed that hypothermia was induced

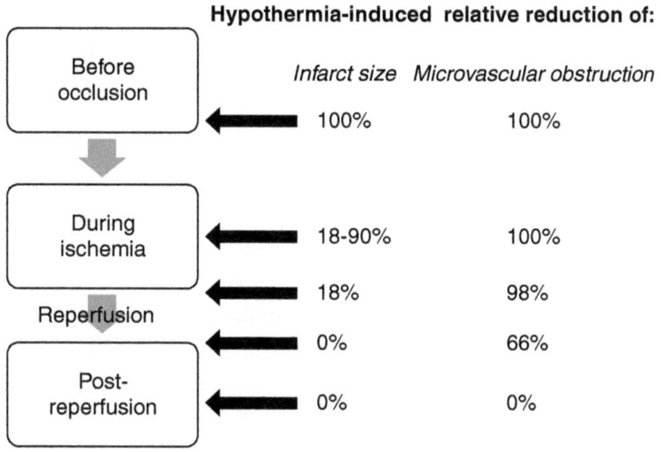

Fig. 11.1 Optimal timing of hypothermia for STEMI-treatment. Relative reduction in infarct size and microvascular obstruction by hypothermia depending on when hypothermia is achieved. The values are estimations based on different animal experiments (see text for references)

more rapidly with a combination of a rapid saline infusion together with endovascular cooling [39]. All patients in the PCI+hypothermia group reached a temperature <35°C before reperfusion. This trial demonstrated that rapidly induced hypothermia was feasible and safe, and that the size of the infarct was significantly reduced (by 38%) [39]. Overall, hypothermia was well tolerated and troponin levels were also significantly reduced. Reperfusion was only delayed by 3 min, which is the time required for an experienced interventionist to insert an endovascular catheter into the vena cava via the femoral vein.

There was a trend towards fewer incidences of heart failure in the PCI+hypothermia group, but also a trend towards more episodes of pneumonia. It is well known that hypothermia increases the risk of infection by inhibiting the immune system, and the prolonged post-reperfusion hypothermia period of 3 h plus 3 h re-warming could increase the risk of lung infections as a result of immobilization and prolonged sedation of the patient.

Analysis of the Pooled Results of the ICE-IT and RAPID MI-ICE Trials

We performed a pooled post-hoc analysis of the results obtained in the two clinical trials, ICE-IT and RAPID MI-ICE (Erlinge et al., submitted). Only patients treated per protocol, and who had undergone infarct size determination with SPECT or cardiac MRI, were included in the analysis.

Compared with the controls (i.e. those receiving PCI only, n=103), the group that was also subjected to hypothermia (n=94), showed a significant 24% reduction in infarct size, expressed as a percentage of the area of the left ventricular myocardium. Among the hypothermia-treated patients in whom a core temperature below 35°C was achieved before reperfusion, the infarct size was reduced by 37% (P=0.01). The benefit observed was similar for both anterior (33% reduction; P=0.03) and inferior infarcts (42% reduction; P=0.04). Although not significant, a similar trend was seen in patients treated with hypothermia when divided according to duration of symptoms: less than 4 h (reduced by 19%, p=0.15), and 4–6 h (reduced by 33%, p=0.07).

The following conclusions can thus be drawn from the analysis of the pooled results:

1. Reaching a temperature of less than 35°C before reperfusion is of paramount importance in reducing the size of the infarct in the treatment of STEMI patients;
2. Hypothermia gives similar benefit in anterior and inferior infarcts, and that
3. Hypothermia seems to be beneficial up to 6 h from the onset of symptoms

Ongoing Clinical Trials

As a follow-up to COOL-MI, COOL-MI 2 used a larger endovascular catheter to provide more rapid cooling. Hypothermia treatment was also started earlier in the emergency room in order to reach a temperature below 35°C before reperfusion. However, the study was terminated due to insufficient funding after 40 patients of the expected 225 had been treated. A trend towards reduced CK-MB has been reported in presentations.

Automated peritoneal lavage with the Velomedix system using cold saline is being used in the CAMARO trial. A European feasibility trial is ongoing with the aim of recruiting 20-100 STEMI patients and applying hypothermia for 3–12 h (ClinicalTrials.gov identifier: NCT01016236). A corkscrew-like device is used to make a hole in the abdomen close to the navel of the conscious patient. However, bleeding could be a problem in STEMI patients, as they are normally heavily treated with anti-coagulants and platelet inhibitors.

The TTM (Target Temperature Management) trial is a randomized clinical trial with target temperatures of 33°C and 36°C for patients with cardiac arrest to limit cerebral injury; the cooling method is optional (ClinicalTrials.gov identifier: NCT01020916). The primary endpoint is all-cause mortality, but a sub-study is being performed in which infarct size is being determined in relation to the area at risk using cardiac MRI, in patients with STEMI as the underlying cause of cardiac arrest. The number of patients expected in the sub-study is 40–50. Previous post-hoc analysis of a subset of 111 patients with cardiac arrest and STEMI in the Hypothermia After Cardiac Arrest (HACA) trial showed reduced CK-MB levels in patients who achieved the target temperature within 8 h of cardiac arrest, but not after 8 h [40].

The CHILL-MI Trial

Based on our animal experiments with the pig model and the RAPID MI-ICE safety & feasibility trial, we concluded that a combination of rapid endovascular cooling and cold saline infusion is a possible way of achieving therapeutic temperatures before reperfusion, with only little delay in reperfusion (3 min).

Based on these findings we designed and recently started the CHILL-MI trial (ClinicalTrials.gov identifier: NCT01379261) using endovascular cooling combined with rapid infusion of up to 2 L cold saline, including both anterior and large inferior STEMI, with up to 6 h of symptoms prior to inclusion. The trial will include 120 patients at 10 international hospitals, and the myocardium at risk and infarct size will be measured after 4 days and 6 months with cardiac MRI. Hypothermia will be maintained for only 1 h after reperfusion, followed by spontaneous re-warming.

One of the advantages of this short cooling protocol is that the whole cooling procedure can be performed in the PCI department, and the endovascular catheter can be removed before the patient is returned to the coronary care unit, thereby excluding the need for treatment in expensive and over-crowded intensive care units. Other advantages of short cooling post-reperfusion are improved patient comfort and possibly a reduced risk of pulmonary infections.

Cooling the Conscious Patient

Most clinical experience of hypothermia has been obtained from cooling unconscious, anesthetized and ventilated patients, either during surgery or after cardiac arrest. Cooling in these situations is more rapid and easier to maintain, because the re-warming/shivering response is abolished. Additional muscle relaxants can be given if required to totally obliterate shivering. In fact, the body temperature of these patients falls spontaneously. Cooling the conscious patient is much more difficult. As the body temperature falls the temperature-controlling center in the brain stem triggers thermoregulatory defenses and powerful re-warming mechanisms. Skin circulation is reduced to maintain core temperature and shivering is initiated. There seems to be a shivering threshold at around 35–36°C, where shivering is most strongly activated. Below this temperature shivering becomes less intense. Once shivering has become fully activated, it is almost impossible to cool the patient. The most important background factors which determine the speed of cooling of the conscious patient are age and weight. Elderly patients have a much weaker shivering response, which facilitates cooling, while overweight patients have a larger body mass, which takes longer to cool.

Experience has shown that there are ways of fooling the body's temperature sensors. Most of the temperature sensors are located in the skin and are strong triggers of shivering. Therefore, surface cooling should be avoided. When using endovascular cooling and intravenous saline infusions, it is possible to fool the skin's temperature sensors by surface counter-warming, either with blankets or more advanced surface warming, such as a Bair Hugger®. A 4°C increase in skin temperature compensates for a 1°C decrease in core temperature [41]. A conscious patient undergoing endovascular cooling and surface warming will/may say that he or she does not feel cold, although their core temperature is 33°C.

Some medication is effective in reducing shivering, especially meperidine (pethidine, demerol). Replacing morphine with meperidine in patients with acute myocardial infarction is very effective (10 mg meperidine is approximately equipotent to 1 mg morphine for pain relief). Meperidine has an almost instant effect on shivering, given in bolus doses of 25–50 mg. Buspirone is given as a tablet (usually 30 mg) and potentiates the anti-shivering effect of meperidine [42]. Other suggested pharmaceutical treatments, such as morphine or alpha-2-receptor agonists, are less effective and it is doubtful whether magnesium has any effect at all.

Hemodynamic Effects of Hypothermia

Deep hypothermia (<30°C) decreases myocardial blood flow, reduces ventricular function and causes spontaneous fibrillation [43]. However, these problems are not apparent during mild hypothermia. Clinical experience shows that cardiac output decreases during mild hypothermia, but this is caused by a reduction in systemic metabolism and the associated reduced demand for cardiac output. At 32°C cardiac output is decreased by 30–40%, but the metabolism is reduced by 50–65%, which gives a net improvement in the balance between supply and demand [44]. Hypothermia causes a decrease in heart rate, most often resulting in a stable heart rate of 50–60 beats/minute. In the normal beating heart, mild hypothermia exerts a positive inotropic effect both *in vitro* [45–47], and *in vivo* [48, 49], but may cause mild diastolic dysfunction [47, 50]. Indeed, hypothermia may even improve hemodynamics in acute cardiogenic shock (see below) [51].

Myocardial perfusion is improved during mild core hypothermia in conscious humans [52]. The peripheral resistance, especially in the skin circulation, increases. Generally, the mean arterial pressure is unchanged, while there is a slight reduction in systolic blood pressure, accompanied by a slight increase in diastolic blood pressure. The kidney perfusion and atrial natriuretic levels increase and antidiuretic hormone levels decrease resulting in "cold diuresis", which if not remedied will result in hypovolemia [44]. However, overall mild hypothermia usually stabilizes the circulation.

Side Effects of Hypothermia

Immunosuppression

Hypothermia causes immunosuppresion by impairing neutrophil and macrophage function and leukocyte migration [44]. The risk of pneumonia may increase, as was seen in the stroke trial ICTUS [53]. However, in the HACA and Bernard trials on cardiac arrest, no increase in infection was seen in the hypothermia groups [1, 2].

Coagulation and Platelet Function

The coagulation system is inhibited by hypothermia, at least at temperatures <34°C [44]. It has been suggested that platelets are also inhibited by hypothermia, and there are some studies supporting this notion [54–56]. However, there are more recent reports suggesting increased platelet reactivity during mild hypothermia [57–60]. We examined platelet activity at 33°C and 37°C and found unchanged or slightly increased platelet activity for most agonists [61]. Interestingly, a resistance to the ADP inhibitor clopidogrel was induced, possibly due to increased sensitivity to ADP activation [61].

The treatment of cardiac arrest patients with hypothermia in the clinical setting has not revealed bleeding complications to be a major problem. Our recommendation for treating cooled STEMI patients is to be very observant not to overdose anticoagulants such as heparins or bivalirudin, and to give antiplatelet therapy as usual.

Metabolism

Increased fat metabolism leads to increased levels of glycerol, free fatty acids and lactate in the blood, which cause mild metabolic acidosis during long periods of hypothermia. Insulin secretion is reduced and together with a relative insulin resistance this may result in increased glucose levels [44, 62].

Ion Changes

Hypothermia induces hypokalemia after a long period of treatment [44]. It is important not to over-compensate this with potassium infusions, since the condition will be reversed upon re-warming.

Arrhythmia

Electrocardiographic changes induced by hypothermia include prolonged PR intervals, increased QT intervals and widening of the QRS complex [44]. Mild hypothermia does not increase the risk of arrhythmia. Indeed, mild hypothermia increases membrane stability and decreases the risk of arrhythmia. However, more severe hypothermia, below 28°C, can increase the risk of arrhythmia and cause spontaneous ventricular fibrillation. In addition, such arrhythmia is more difficult to treat, as the myocardium is less responsive to antiarrhythmic drugs. The risk of ventricular fibrillation is reduced by the stabilization of cardiomyocyte membranes during mild hypothermia [63]. Mild hypothermia (33°C) has been shown to improve the success of defibrillation compared with normothermia, with an increased chance of achieving return of spontaneous circulation (ROSC) [64]. More severe hypothermia (30°C) has been found to facilitate transthoracic defibrillation in a swine model, while moderate hypothermia (33°C) did not alter the energy required for defibrillation [65]. Since impedance increases and current falls during hypothermia, the improved shock success is due to a hypothermia-induced change in the mechanical or electrophysiological properties of the myocardium [65].

Cardiogenic Shock

Even patients experiencing cardiogenic shock have a good outcome after treatment with hypothermia [66]. We examined the effects of hypothermia in a pig model of cardiogenic shock [51]. Cooling one group of pigs to <34°C resulted in better survival; five out of eight pigs in the normothermia group died, while all pigs in the hypothermia group survived (n=8). Stroke volume and blood pressure were maintained at a higher level in the hypothermia group, whereas the heart rate was significantly lower. Cardiac output did not differ between the groups. Blood gas analysis revealed higher mixed venous oxygen saturation, pH, and base excess in the hypothermia group, indicating less metabolic acidosis [51].

In a model of resuscitated pigs, Schwarzl and coworkers used pressure–volume analysis and found improved left ventricular (LV) systolic function during mild hypothermia, but also demonstrated decreased LV end-diastolic distensibility [50]. Mild hypothermia did not increase plasma catecholamine levels, and spectral analysis of heart rate variability revealed reduced sympathetic activation. They concluded that mild hypothermia after cardiac resuscitation improves systolic myocardial function without further sympathetic activation. Reduced metabolism during hypothermia has been reported to outweigh the decreased in CO and to thus act favorably on the balance between systemic oxygen supply and demand [50].

In summary, hypothermia reduces acute mortality in cardiogenic shock models, improves hemodynamic parameters and reduces metabolic acidosis. These findings suggest a possible clinical benefit of therapeutic hypothermia for patients with acute cardiogenic shock.

Conclusions

In conclusion, mild hypothermia may be of benefit as an adjunctive treatment for STEMI as it has positive effects on the four components of ischemia reperfusion injury: myocardial stunning, microvascular obstruction, reperfusion arrhythmia and lethal reperfusion injury. Hypothermia could be clinically used to treat cardiogenic shock, which still has a mortality rate of nearly 50%, or to stabilize the circulation during septic shock. Rapid initiation of hypothermia in the field could improve ROSC in patients with cardiac arrest resulting from ventricular arrhythmia.

For cardiac protection, evidence suggests that therapeutic hypothermia should be instigated as early as possible during ischemia, at least before reperfusion. Continued treatment after reperfusion can probably be relatively short. Hypothermia has wide-ranging effects on most of the mechanisms involved in ischemia and reperfusion injury, which may explain the potent, highly reproducible cardioprotective effects seen in a multitude of studies in different species. Cooling conscious patients with STEMI is safe, feasible and well tolerated, but anti-shivering strategies must be employed. Clinical results indicate that achieving a core temperature of less than 35°C before reperfusion is of paramount importance in order to reduce the extent of the infarct in the treatment of STEMI patients. Larger clinical studies such as the CHILL-MI trial are ongoing.

Disclosures The author received endovascular cooling catheters and funding for MRI examinations in the RAPID MI-ICE study from InnerCool Therapies, now Philips Healthcare.

References

1. Bernard SA, Gray TW, Buist MD, et al. Treatment of comatose survivors of out-of-hospital cardiac arrest with induced hypothermia. N Engl J Med. 2002; 346(8):557–63.
2. Hypothermia after Cardiac Arrest Study Group. Mild therapeutic hypothermia to improve the neurologic outcome after cardiac arrest. N Engl J Med. 2002; 346(8):549–56.
3. Braunwald E, Antman EM, Beasley JW, et al. ACC/AHA guideline update for the management of patients with unstable angina and non-ST-segment elevation myocardial infarction–2002: summary article: a report of the American College of Cardiology/American Heart Association Task Force on Practice Guidelines (Committee on the Management of Patients With Unstable Angina). Circulation. 2002;106(14):1893–900.
4. Varon J, Acosta P. Therapeutic hypothermia: past, present, and future. Chest. 2008;133(5):1267–74.
5. Tissier R, Chenoune M, Ghaleh B, et al. The small chill: mild hypothermia for cardioprotection? Cardiovasc Res. 2011;88(3):406–14.
6. Hale SL, Kloner RA. Mild hypothermia as a cardioprotective approach for acute myocardial infarction: laboratory to clinical application. J Cardiovasc Pharmacol Ther. 2011;16(2):131–9.
7. Gotberg M, Olivecrona GK, Engblom H, et al. Rapid short-duration hypothermia with cold saline and endovascular cooling before reperfusion reduces microvascular obstruction and myocardial infarct size. BMC Cardiovasc Disord. 2008;8:7.
8. Miller TD, Christian TF, Hopfenspirger MR, et al. Infarct size after acute myocardial infarction measured by quantitative tomographic 99mTc sestamibi imaging predicts subsequent mortality. Circulation. 1995;92(3):334–41.
9. Burns RJ, Gibbons RJ, Yi Q, et al. The relationships of left ventricular ejection fraction, end-systolic volume index and infarct size to six-month mortality after hospital discharge following myocardial infarction treated by thrombolysis. J Am Coll Cardiol. 2002;39(1):30–6.
10. Kloner RA. Does reperfusion injury exist in humans? J Am Coll Cardiol. 1993;21(2):537–45.
11. Ambrosio G, Tritto II. Lethal myocardial reperfusion injury: does it exist, should we treat it? J Thromb Thrombolysis. 1997;4(1):69–70.
12. Kloner RA, Ganote CE, Jennings RB. The "no-reflow" phenomenon after temporary coronary occlusion in the dog. J Clin Invest. 1974;54(6):1496–508.
13. Yellon DM, Hausenloy DJ. Myocardial reperfusion injury. N Engl J Med. 2007;357(11):1121–35.
14. O'Neill WW, Dixon SR, Grines CL. The year in interventional cardiology. J Am Coll Cardiol. 2005; 45(7):1117–34.
15. Grines CL. Intravascular cooling adjunctive to percutaneous coronary intervention for acute myocardial infarction. Presented at transcatheter cardiovascular therapeutics. Washington DC; 2004.
16. O' Neill WW. Cooling as an adjunct to primary PCI for myocardial infarction. Presented at transcatheter cardiovascular therapeutics. Washington DC; 2004.
17. Abendschein DR, Tacker Jr WA, Babbs CF. Protection of ischemic myocardium by whole-body hypothermia after coronary artery occlusion in dogs. Am Heart J. 1978;96(6):772–80.

18. Chien GL, Wolff RA, Davis RF, et al. "Normothermic range" temperature affects myocardial infarct size. Cardiovasc Res. 1994;28(7):1014–7.
19. Duncker DJ, Klassen CL, Ishibashi Y, et al. Effect of temperature on myocardial infarction in swine. Am J Physiol. 1996;270(4 Pt 2):H1189–99.
20. Hale SL, Kloner RA. Elevated body temperature during myocardial ischemia/reperfusion exacerbates necrosis and worsens no-reflow. Coron Artery Dis. 2002;13(3):177–81.
21. Hale SL, Dave RH, Kloner RA. Regional hypothermia reduces myocardial necrosis even when instituted after the onset of ischemia. Basic Res Cardiol. 1997;92(5):351–7.
22. Hale SL, Kloner RA. Myocardial temperature in acute myocardial infarction: protection with mild regional hypothermia. Am J Physiol. 1997;273(1 Pt 2):H220–7.
23. Hale SL, Kloner RA. Myocardial temperature reduction attenuates necrosis after prolonged ischemia in rabbits. Cardiovasc Res. 1998;40(3):502–7.
24. Tissier R, Couvreur N, Ghaleh B, et al. Rapid cooling preserves the ischaemic myocardium against mitochondrial damage and left ventricular dysfunction. Cardiovasc Res. 2009;83(2):345–53.
25. Dave RH, Hale SL, Kloner RA. Hypothermic, closed circuit pericardioperfusion: a potential cardioprotective technique in acute regional ischemia. J Am Coll Cardiol. 1998;31(7):1667–71.
26. Otake H, Shite J, Paredes OL, et al. Catheter-based transcoronary myocardial hypothermia attenuates arrhythmia and myocardial necrosis in pigs with acute myocardial infarction. J Am Coll Cardiol. 2007;49(2): 250–60.
27. Wakida Y, Haendchen RV, Kobayashi S, et al. Percutaneous cooling of ischemic myocardium by hypothermic retroperfusion of autologous arterial blood: effects on regional myocardial temperature distribution and infarct size. J Am Coll Cardiol. 1991; 18(1):293–300.
28. Maeng M, Mortensen UM, Kristensen J, et al. Hypothermia during reperfusion does not reduce myocardial infarct size in pigs. Basic Res Cardiol. 2006;101(1):61–8.
29. Dae MW, Gao DW, Sessler DI, et al. Effect of endovascular cooling on myocardial temperature, infarct size, and cardiac output in human-sized pigs. Am J Physiol Heart Circ Physiol. 2002;282(5):H1584–91.
30. Dixon SR, Whitbourn RJ, Dae MW, et al. Induction of mild systemic hypothermia with endovascular cooling during primary percutaneous coronary intervention for acute myocardial infarction. J Am Coll Cardiol. 2002;40(11):1928–34.
31. Kandzari DE, Chu A, Brodie BR, et al. Feasibility of endovascular cooling as an adjunct to primary percutaneous coronary intervention (results of the LOWTEMP pilot study). Am J Cardiol. 2004; 93(5):636–9.
32. Ly HQ, Denault A, Dupuis J, et al. A pilot study: the Noninvasive Surface Cooling Thermoregulatory System for Mild Hypothermia Induction in Acute Myocardial Infarction (the NICAMI Study). Am Heart J. 2005;150(5):933.
33. Gotberg M, van der Pals J, Olivecrona GK, et al. Optimal timing of hypothermia in relation to myocardial reperfusion. Basic Res Cardiol. 2011;106(5): 697–708.
34. Jaffe R, Charron T, Puley G, et al. Microvascular obstruction and the no-reflow phenomenon after percutaneous coronary intervention. Circulation. 2008; 117(24):3152–6.
35. Lima JA, Judd RM, Bazille A, et al. Regional heterogeneity of human myocardial infarcts demonstrated by contrast-enhanced MRI. Potential mechanisms. Circulation. 1995;92(5):1117–25.
36. Wu KC, Zerhouni EA, Judd RM, et al. Prognostic significance of microvascular obstruction by magnetic resonance imaging in patients with acute myocardial infarction. Circulation. 1998;97(8):765–72.
37. Choi CJ, Haji-Momenian S, Dimaria JM, et al. Infarct involution and improved function during healing of acute myocardial infarction: the role of microvascular obstruction. J Cardiovasc Magn Reson. 2004;6(4): 917–25.
38. Hale SL, Dae MW, Kloner RA. Hypothermia during reperfusion limits 'no-reflow' injury in a rabbit model of acute myocardial infarction. Cardiovasc Res. 2003; 59(3):715–22.
39. Gotberg M, Olivecrona GK, Koul S, et al. A pilot study of rapid cooling by cold saline and endovascular cooling before reperfusion in patients with ST-elevation myocardial infarction. Circ Cardiovasc Interv. 2010;3(5):400–7.
40. Koreny M, Sterz F, Uray T, et al. Effect of cooling after human cardiac arrest on myocardial infarct size. Resuscitation. 2009;80(1):56–60.
41. Cheng C, Matsukawa T, Sessler DI, et al. Increasing mean skin temperature linearly reduces the core-temperature thresholds for vasoconstriction and shivering in humans. Anesthesiology. 1995;82(5):1160–8.
42. Mokhtarani M, Mahgoub AN, Morioka N, et al. Buspirone and meperidine synergistically reduce the shivering threshold. Anesth Analg. 2001;93(5):1233–9.
43. Tveita T, Mortensen E, Hevroy O, et al. Experimental hypothermia: effects of core cooling and rewarming on hemodynamics, coronary blood flow, and myocardial metabolism in dogs. Anesth Analg. 1994; 79(2):212–8.
44. Polderman KH. Mechanisms of action, physiological effects, and complications of hypothermia. Crit Care Med. 2009;37(7 Suppl):S186–202.
45. Kusuoka H, Ikoma Y, Futaki S, et al. Positive inotropism in hypothermia partially depends on an increase in maximal Ca(2+)-activated force. Am J Physiol. 1991;261(4 Pt 2):H1005–10.
46. Suga H, Goto Y, Igarashi Y, et al. Cardiac cooling increases Emax without affecting relation between O_2 consumption and systolic pressure-volume area in dog left ventricle. Circ Res. 1988;63(1):61–71.
47. Weisser J, Martin J, Bisping E, et al. Influence of mild hypothermia on myocardial contractility and

circulatory function. Basic Res Cardiol. 2001;96(2): 198–205.
48. Nishimura Y, Naito Y, Nishioka T, et al. The effects of cardiac cooling under surface-induced hypothermia on the cardiac function in the in situ heart. Interact Cardiovasc Thorac Surg. 2005;4(2):101–5.
49. Post H, Schmitto JD, Steendijk P, et al. Cardiac function during mild hypothermia in pigs: increased inotropy at the expense of diastolic dysfunction. Acta Physiol (Oxf). 2010;199(1):43–52.
50. Schwarzl M, Steendijk P, Huber S, et al. The induction of mild hypothermia improves systolic function of the resuscitated porcine heart at no further sympathetic activation. Acta Physiol (Oxf). 2011;203: 409–18.
51. Gotberg M, van der Pals J, Olivecrona GK, et al. Mild hypothermia reduces acute mortality and improves hemodynamic outcome in a cardiogenic shock pig model. Resuscitation. 2010;81(9):1190–6.
52. Frank SM, Satitpunwaycha P, Bruce SR, et al. Increased myocardial perfusion and sympathoadrenal activation during mild core hypothermia in awake humans. Clin Sci (Lond). 2003;104(5):503–8.
53. Hemmen TM, Raman R, Guluma KZ, et al. Intravenous thrombolysis plus hypothermia for acute treatment of ischemic stroke (ICTuS-L): final results. Stroke. 2010;41(10):2265–70.
54. Frelinger 3rd AL, Furman MI, Barnard MR, et al. Combined effects of mild hypothermia and glycoprotein IIb/IIIa antagonists on platelet-platelet and leukocyte-platelet aggregation. Am J Cardiol. 2003;92(9): 1099–101.
55. Michelson AD, MacGregor H, Barnard MR, et al. Reversible inhibition of human platelet activation by hypothermia in vivo and in vitro. Thromb Haemost. 1994;71(5):633–40.
56. Michelson AD, Barnard MR, Khuri SF, et al. The effects of aspirin and hypothermia on platelet function in vivo. Br J Haematol. 1999;104(1):64–8.
57. Lindenblatt N, Menger MD, Klar E, et al. Sustained hypothermia accelerates microvascular thrombus formation in mice. Am J Physiol Heart Circ Physiol. 2005;289(6):H2680–7.
58. Xavier RG, White AE, Fox SC, et al. Enhanced platelet aggregation and activation under conditions of hypothermia. Thromb Haemost. 2007;98(6):1266–75.
59. Scharbert G, Kalb M, Marschalek C, et al. The effects of test temperature and storage temperature on platelet aggregation: a whole blood in vitro study. Anesth Analg. 2006;102(4):1280–4.
60. Zhang JN, Wood J, Bergeron AL, et al. Effects of low temperature on shear-induced platelet aggregation and activation. J Trauma. 2004;57(2):216–23.
61. Hogberg C, Erlinge D, Braun OO. Mild hypothermia does not attenuate platelet aggregation and may even increase ADP-stimulated platelet aggregation after clopidogrel treatment. Thromb J. 2009;7:2.
62. Lehot JJ, Piriz H, Villard J, et al. Glucose homeostasis comparison between hypothermic and normothermic cardiopulmonary bypass. Chest. 1992;102(1): 106–11.
63. Harada M, Honjo H, Yamazaki M, et al. Moderate hypothermia increases the chance of spiral wave collision in favor of self-termination of ventricular tachycardia/fibrillation. Am J Physiol Heart Circ Physiol. 2008;294(4):H1896–905.
64. Boddicker KA, Zhang Y, Zimmerman MB, et al. Hypothermia improves defibrillation success and resuscitation outcomes from ventricular fibrillation. Circulation. 2005;111(24):3195–201.
65. Rhee BJ, Zhang Y, Boddicker KA, et al. Effect of hypothermia on transthoracic defibrillation in a swine model. Resuscitation. 2005;65(1):79–85.
66. Hovdenes J, Laake JH, Aaberge L, et al. Therapeutic hypothermia after out-of-hospital cardiac arrest: experiences with patients treated with percutaneous coronary intervention and cardiogenic shock. Acta Anaesthesiol Scand. 2007;51(2):137–42.

Index

J.B. Lundbye (ed.), *Therapeutic Hypothermia After Cardiac Arrest*,
DOI 10.1007/978-1-4471-2951-6, © Springer-Verlag London 2012

MIX
Papier aus verantwortungsvollen Quellen
Paper from responsible sources
FSC® C105338

If you have any concerns about our products,
you can contact us on
ProductSafety@springernature.com

In case Publisher is established outside the EU,
the EU authorized representative is:
Springer Nature Customer Service Center GmbH
Europaplatz 3, 69115 Heidelberg, Germany

Printed by Libri Plureos GmbH
in Hamburg, Germany